Praise for 2004 edition of
The Good Euthanasia Guide

"The book is not a 'how-to' manual, but one that points people towards the countries and organizations that will assist a death."
— The Guardian, London

"He writes authoritatively on the social history of the movement in the United States, the split with Dr. Kevorkian, and the political struggles in Oregon and Maine."
—

"It's mood is unsensational and its
a stimulus for the newcomer to the
peaceful death, and also for the seasoned campaigner."
— World Right To Die Newsletter

"Inspired by guide books for the discerning consumer."
— Reuters newsagency

"Finally, here, in one convenient place, are all the facts and history of our movement — all presented in a clear, direct manner, as you would expect from such brilliant journalist."
— Arizona End-of-Life Choices newsletter

"It has been written from the head and the heart of a man who 'was there,' quite possibly more so than anyone could claim to have been."
— Free To Go, Canada

"The book is not a 'how-to' like 'Final Exit' but a 'where-to' such has never been published before."
— Friends At The End newsletter, Scotland

"A controversial new book [which] has the sole intention of teaching people the so-called 'do's and don'ts' of ending their own lives."
— Family News in Focus

The Good Euthanasia Guide

Derek Humphry

2006

Books by Derek Humphry

Because They're Black, 1971
(Martin Luther King Memorial Prize, 1972)

Police Power and Black People, 1972

Passports and Politics, 1974

The Cricket Conspiracy, 1975

False Messiah (with David Tindall), 1977

Policing The Police (with Peter Hain), 1979

Jean's Way, 1978

Let Me Die Before I Wake, 1981

The Right to Die (with Ann Wickett), 1986

Final Exit, 1991
(2nd edition 1997, 3rd edition 2003)

Dying With Dignity, 1992

Freedom To Die (with Mary Clement), 1998

The Good
Euthanasia
Guide

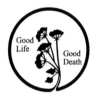

Derek Humphry

A Norris Lane Press original paperback

2006 new printing, updated

Published by the Norris Lane Press/ERGO
24829 Norris Lane
Junction City OR 97448 USA
<*derekhumphry@starband.net*>

THE GOOD EUTHANASIA GUIDE

First Norris Lane Press edition published 2004.

Design and jacket by Tracy Reith
Digitally printed by Berryville Graphics, Virginia

ISBN 978-0-9768283-1-0
Library of Congress Catalog Number 2004366647

ISBN 978-0-9768283-1-0

51400

9 780976 828310

Acknowledgement
*My thanks to Faye Girsh—a doughty
campaigner for choice in dying—for her valuable
contributions to this book.*

*"Death does not always come at the right time.
I believe there are conditions under which I would
prefer not to live, situations where
I would be better off dead."*
— Prof. John Hartwig, philosopher

*"Those who come after us will wonder why we
kept a human being alive against his own will when we
would have been punished by the State if we kept an
animal alive under similar conditions."*
— Rev. Leslie Weatherhead

*"Choice in the manner of our dying is
the ultimate civil liberty."*
— Derek Humphry

*"Better the cup of hemlock in time.
Why nurse disease or deformity? Death is not an
evil, but vileness is; when vileness is cultivated for
the sake of life it renders life vile also."*
— George Santayana

*"Assisted suicide should never be a requirement, but
it should always be a legal and moral option."*
— Bishop John Shelby Spong

CONTENTS

Definitions of words and terms as used in this book

Choices in dying = Making a commonsense decision on the options for how you will die.

Right-to-die = Choice in the manner of dying (generic).

Euthanasia = Help with a good death (generic).

Passive euthanasia = Disconnection of life-support equipment leading to death.

Voluntary euthanasia = Death by lethal injection by doctor as requested by patient.

Involuntary euthanasia = Doctor ends life of comatose patient to end hopeless suffering.

Assisted suicide = Person/s helping terminal patient to die at his/her request.

Physician-assisted suicide = Doctor prescribes lethal overdose which patient can choose to drink.

Non physician-assisted suicide = Term used mainly in Switzerland where most assisted suicides are by trained volunteers, rarely by doctors.

Suicide = Killing oneself. In Christian theology, self-murder or *felo de se.*

Silent suicide = Starving oneself to death.

Mercy killing = Taking the life of another in the belief that this is a compassionate act because the ill person is unable to.

Rational suicide = Killing oneself for a considered, logical reason.

Self-deliverance = Killing oneself to escape the continued suffering of a terminal or hopeless illness.

Terminal illness = The condition of a person who is beyond medical help and will die shortly. The hospice movement usually says about six months left to live.

Hopelessly ill = A person whose degenerative illness is irreversible and has severely limited quality of life.

Terms such as *'physician aid-in-dying'* and *'physician-assisted dying'* (PAD) are too euphemistic and vague for use in this book. Nevertheless, some people like them exactly because they are gentler words. But they can lead to misunderstandings.

PREFACE

The Good Food Guide, the Good Hotel Guide, the Good Pub Guide, and so forth, are now all staples of reference literature to help make our lives more congenial. Just as surely as we need to eat, sleep and drink right, it is also certain that we will some day die. So why not some advanced research to get that right, too?

This is not a 'how-to' book like my *'Final Exit'* but a 'where-to' and 'who.' *The Good Euthanasia Guide* is not about death, funerals or grieving. The book is concerned with making a conscious, ethical, and common sense plan about dying—which, according to your medical fortune, can take years, months, days or minutes.

Don't bother to acquire this book if you are a person who believes that a religious deity is in sole charge of your life and dying.

As well as names and contact details of groups worldwide which attempt to ensure that the final episode of a person's life is carried out with dignity, compassion, and self-control, it helps to be aware of the recent history the right-to-choose-to-die movement.

An understanding of the rise and fall of that eccentric messiah, Dr. Jack Kevorkian, and the roller-coaster progress of the Hemlock Society (now dissolved into another organization) help define the issues for a newcomer to the subject.

As the lives of new generations begin to run their courses, a peek at what the future may hold for voluntary euthanasia may also be instructive. The debate has already begun on whether the very old, in frail health, may choose to hasten their ends, perhaps with help. And do people with protracted, untreatable mental agony deserve help to die? Let the debate begin.

D.H.

A GUIDE TO RIGHT-TO-DIE GROUPS IN THE WORLD

Membership fees for the organizations are omitted. Some groups are not membership organizations but rely on donations and legacies. Generally, the membership fee is around $40 US for a couple and $30 for an individual. Most groups also allow discounts for the needy and for seniors.

Australia

EXIT International
(formerly EXIT Australia/New Zealand)
PO Box 37781
Winnellie
Northern Territory 0821

Phone: 0500-83-1929
   Fax: 08-8983-2949
 Email: exit@euthanasia.net
   Web: www.exitinternational.net

Founded: 1998. The most progressive group in the southern hemisphere and perhaps the world. Its chief, Dr. Philip Nitschke, believes everybody who wishes to end their life should have the opportunity to do so. The group gives 'euthanasia workshops' throughout the country. It is ceaselessly working for new ways in which dying people can self-deliver without a doctor and without breaking the law.

Northern Territory Voluntary Euthanasia Society
GPO Box 2734
Darwin
Northern Territory 0801

Phone: +61 8-8927-2294
   Fax: +61 8-8927-2294
 Email: ntves@bigpond.com.au

Founded 1995 in the wake of the unexpected legislation of voluntary euthanasia in the territory. The Federal Government repealed the law in 1997.

South Australia Voluntary Euthanasia Society
PO Box 2151
Kent Town
South Australia 5071

Phone: 8-8265-3548
   Fax: 8-8265-2287
 Email: info@saves.asn.au

Founded 1983. Mission: Chiefly lobbying for legislative change.

Voluntary Euthanasia Society of New South Wales, Inc.
PO Box 25
Broadway
New South Wales 2007

Email: mail@vesnsw.org.au
  Web: www.vesnsw.org.au

Founded 1983. The aim of the Voluntary Euthanasia Society of NSW is to promote legislation which, with the proper safeguards, entitles any person suffering severe pain or distress, with no reasonable prospect of recovery, to a painless, medically assisted and dignified death in accordance with his or her expressed direction.

Voluntary Euthanasia Society of Queensland
PO Box 424
Mount Gravatt
Brisbane
Queensland 4122

Phone: 61-500-858-500
 Email: raysan@optusnet.com.au
  Web: www.connectqld.org.au/vesq

Voluntary Euthanasia Society of Tasmania
PO Box 1022
Sandy Bay
Tasmania 7006

Phone: +03 6234 1425
        +03 6244 3821
 Email: hcutts@netspace.net.au
  Web: www.tased.edu.au/tasonline/vest

Promotes legislation that gives effect to freedom of choice and individual human rights, so that any person suffering, through illness or disability, severe pain or distress for which no remedy is available that is acceptable to the person, should be entitled by law to a painless and dignified death in accordance with his or her express direction. Provides individual counselling. To pursue actively a continuing public education policy to achieve such legislation.

Dying With Dignity, Victoria
3/98 Salisbury Avenue
Blackburn, Victoria 3130

Phone: 61-3-987-7677
Email: vesv@vesv.org.au
Web: www.vesv.org.au

Founded 1974. Mission: Promoting legislation to enable incurably ill people to choose a painless and dignified death. Dying with Dignity (formerly VESV) is not able to help people end their lives.

Voluntary Euthanasia Society of West Australia
PO Box 7243
Cloisters Square
Perth
West Australia 6850

Phone: 9276-9144
Fax: 9381-1893
Email: info@waves.org.au
Web: www.waves.org.au

Founded 1980. Mission: "To bring about such changes to Western Australian Statute Law and to medical ethics as will allow a person, suffering severe pain or distress with no reasonable prospect of recovery, to receive, with the proper safeguards, a painless medically assisted and dignified death in accordance with his or her expressed wishes."

Belgium

Recht op Waardig Sterven
(Flemish-speaking. Known as RWS)
Constitutiestraat 33,
B-2060 Antwerpen

Phone: 32-3-272-5163
Fax: 32-3-272-5163
Email: info@rws.be
Web: www.rws.be

Founded 1983.

Association pour le Droit de Mourir dans la Dignite
(French speaking. Known as ADMD)
55 Rue du Président
B-1050 Bruxelles

Phone: 32-2-502-0485
Fax: 32-2-502-6150
Email: info@admd.be
Web: http://perso.infonie.be/admd

Founded 1981.

Britain (United Kingdom)

Friends at the End (FATE)
11 Westbourne Gardens
Glasgow G12 9XD

Phone: +0141-334-3287
   Fax: +0141-334-3287
Email: friendsattheend@beeb.net
   Web: www.friends-at-the-end.fsnet.co.uk

A break-away from Scottish EXIT in l995, it is willing to give cautious advice and literature on hastened death of the terminally ill.

EXIT Scotland
17 Hart Street
Edinburgh EH1 3RN

Phone: +131-556-4404
 Email: exit@euthanasia.cc
   Web: www.euthanasia.cc

Founded in l980 by the late Sheila Little, EXIT has gone through many changes and downsizing. It published the first 'how-to' booklet in l981. EXIT supports both self-deliverance and assisted suicide. It works within the law, but by treading a fine line on providing effective information on self-deliverance to members they are able to help people without risking the small organisation's existence by breaking the law.

Dignity in Dying
13 Prince of Wales Terrace
Kensington
London W8 5PG

Phone: 2079-377-770
    Fax: 2073-762-648
  Email: info@ves.org.uk
    Web: www.ves.org.uk

The London group is the oldest of its type in the world (1935) and has fluctuated in its mission. Currently, it concentrates on parliamentary law reform for physician-assisted suicide and promoting Advance Directives. It declines to give any help or advice on hastened death. But it does campaign for people with terminal illnesses to be allowed to ask for medical help to die at a time of their choosing, within proper legal safeguards. It wants to make back-street suicides and 'mercy killings' a thing of the past.

The Voluntary Euthanasia Society of England and Wales officially changed its name in 2005 to "Dignity in Dying." There was a 79% support for this alteration which, by removal of the word 'euthanasia', is hoped to improve its public image.

Canada

Choices in Dying
Box 79521 Kingsway RPO
Vancouver, BC V5R 5Z6

Phone: 604-451-9626
Fax: 604-525-3374
Email: choicesindying@telus.net

Dying With Dignity
55 Eglinton Avenue East, Suite 802
Toronto, Ontario M4P 1G8

Phone: 1-800-495-6156
416-486-3998
Fax: 416-486-5562
Email: info@dyingwithdignity.ca
Web: www.dyingwithdignity.ca

Founded 1980 by the late Marilyn Seguin, DWD is developing into a progressive and strong force for the right-to-die in Canada. Helps members whatever way is possible within the law. Dying With Dignity is a registered charitable society whose mission it is to improve the quality of dying for all Canadians in accordance with their own wishes, values, and beliefs.

Right to Die Society of Canada
145 Macdonell Ave
Toronto, Ontario M6R 2A4

Phone: 416-535-0690
 Email: ruth@righttodie.ca
  Web: www.righttodie.ca

As it does not have charitable status, the Society is able to be active politically. It canvases Members of Parliament for their support on law reform, which is its focus for the future. In addition, it works with people for whom law reform will come too late. It gives them information and support that will let them come as close as possible to dying on their own terms. It hopes that before long it will be able to provide companionship at the time of self-deliverance, for people who choose this option and who have been able to set up an arrangement by which the authorities can satisfy themselves that no law has been broken and no charges need to be laid.

Denmark

EVD (En Vaerdig Dod)
Peters Fabers Vej 37 st th
8210 Arhus V
Denmark

  Web: www.e-v-d.dk

Founded 2000. 300 members. Will host the 2007 Right-to-Die Europe conference in Aarhus.

Colombia

Fundacion Pro Derecho a Morir Dignamente
Carrera 11 No. 73 - 44 officina 508
Bogota, Colombia

Phone: +57-1-345-40-65
 Fax: +57-1-313-16-07
 Email: info@dmd.org.co
  Web: www.dmd.org.co

Founded 1979. Mission: Mainly educational and promoting Living Wills and patients' rights.

Finland

Exitus Ry
Post Box 130
FI-00141 Helsinki
Finland

 Email: maria.marjukka.lehtinen@saunalahi.fi

Advocates Advance Directives now, and seeks to have a law passed allowing active voluntary euthanasia.

Pro Gratia of Helsinki
Laajasalonkaari 15 a
FIN-00840 Helsinki

Phone: +358 9 698-4415
 Fax: +358-9491-292

France

Association pour le Droit de Mourir dans la Dignite (ADMD)
50 rue de Chabrol
75010 Paris

Phone: 48-00-04-16
   Fax: 01-48-00-05-72
  Email: info@admd.net
   Web: www.admd.net

Founded 1980. Mission: legislative reform and education. ADMD had 38,000 members in 2005.

Germany

Deutsche Gesellschaft Fur Humanes Sterben e.V (DGHS)
Lange Gasse 2-4
Postfach 11 05 29
Augsburg 86030

Phone: 49-821-502-350
   Fax: 49-821-502-3555
  Email: info@dghs.de
      dghsaugsb@aol.com
   Web: www.dghs.de

Founded 1980. Mission: Lobbies for law reform, distributes Living Wills, and publishes a colorful newsletter.

India

Society for the Right to Die with Dignity
Nanvarati Hospital
SV Road, Vile Parle (w)
Mumbahai 400 058

Phone: 91-22-618-255
Fax: 91-22-611-9363
Email: nagraj@giasbm01.vsnl.net.in

Israel

LILACH, The Israel Society for the Right to Live and Die With Dignity
PO Box 14409
Tel Aviv 61143

Phone: 972-3-673-0577
Email: lilach19@zahav.net.il
Web: www.lilach.org.il

Founded 1987. Pushes for Living Wills and legislative reform.

Italy

EXIT—Italia
Associazione Italiana per il Diritto ad una Morte Dignitosa
Corso Monte Cucco 144
10141 Torino

Phone: +39 11-770 7126
   Fax: +39 11-770 7126
Email: exit-italia@libero.it
   Web: www.exit-italia.it

Seeking law reform on hastened death.

Libera Uscita
Via Genova 24
00184 Rome

Phone: +39-0637823807
   Fax: +39-0648931008
Email: info@liberauscita.it
         associazioneliberauscita@hotmail.com
   Web: www.liberauscita.it

Libera Uscita is a non-political association founded in Rome with organizational basis all over Italy. Founded in 2000. The aim of the association is to develop the debate on bioethical themes, starting with euthanasia and the right to choose consciously a therapeutical treatment as far as its withhold or withdraw. The association has two draft bills—one on euthanasia, the other on Living Wills—which were recently presented to the Chamber of Deputies and to the Senate.

Japan

Japan Society for Dying With Dignity
Watanabe Building 202, 2-29-1 Hongou
Bunkyo-Ku, Tokyo 113

Phone: 81-3-3818-6563
    Fax: 81-3-3818-6562
  Email: info@songenshi-kyokai.com
    Web: www.songenshi-kyokai.com

Founded l976. Has approx. 100,000 members. Mission:
Education, Living Wills and reforming legislation.

Luxembourg

**Association pour le Droit de Mourir dans la
Dignite (ADMDL)**
37 Route de Longwy
L-4750
Petange
Luxembourg

Phone: 352-594-505
    Fax: 352-2659-0482
  Email: admdl@pt.lu
    Web: admdl.lu

Founded l988. Came close in 2003 to achieving law
reform on euthanasia, losing by a narrow vote.

The Netherlands

Right to Die – NL (formerly NVVE)
Postbus 75331
Leidsegracht 103
1070 AH Amsterdam

Phone: +31 20-620-0690
   Fax: +31 20-420-7216
  Email: euthanasie@nvve.nl
   Web: www.nvve.nl

Founded 1973 and spent 30 years educating and driving for law reform, which succeeded in 2002 legalizing voluntary euthanasia and physician-assisted suicide under strict guidelines. Changed its name in 2003 from NVVE. Has approx. 100,000 members.

New Zealand

Voluntary Euthanasia Society of New Zealand
PO Box 26095
Epsom Auckland 3

Phone: 64-9-630 7035
   Fax: 64-9-630 7035
  Email: ves@clear.net.nz
   Web: www.ves.org.nz

In 1978 euthanasia groups were formed in the north and south islands with the aim of changing the law to allow assisted suicide. Following a narrow defeat in Parliament in 2004, the two societies decided to merge to achieve greater political strength.

Norway

Foreningen Retten til en Verdig Død
Ullern Alle 2
0381 Oslo

Phone: 47 22 73 04 80
 Fax: 47 22 13 32 39
Email: l-livste@online.no
 Web: www.livstestament.org

South Africa

South African Voluntary Euthanasia Society (SAVES)
PO Box 1460
Wandsbeck 3631
KwaZulu, Natal

Phone: 141-334-3287
 Fax: 141-334-3287
Email: livingwill@3ico.za
 Web: www.Livingwill.co.za

Founded 1974. Concentrates on education and distributing Living Wills. Has 46,000 members.

Spain

Derecho a Morir Dignamente (DMD)
Avda.Portal del Angel 7-4 atico B
08002 Barcelona

Phone: 343-412-3203
Email: admd@admd.e.telephonica.net
Web: www.eutanasia.ws

Founded 1984. It is now the umbrella group for four divisions around Spain.

Sweden

Rätten Til Var Död
Höganäsgaten 2 C
735-30 Upsala

Phone: +46 18-104140
Fax: +46 40-964498
Email: appelcomp@tella.com

Founded 1973.

Switzerland

DIGNITAS
Postfach 9
CH 8127 Forch

Phone: +980-44-59
  Fax: +980-14-21
 Email: dignitas@dignitas.ch
  Web: www.dignitas.ch

DIGNITAS is a tiny organization near Zurich that will help terminally ill, chronically ill and sometimes very seriously mentally ill people. Following worldwide publicity in 2003 it virtually had to shut down because of overwhelming work and lack of finance. It resumed operating in 2004.

Exit/ADMD Suisse Romande
C.P. 110
CH 1211 Geneva 17

Phone: +22 735-77-60
  Fax: +22 735-77-65
 Email: info@exit-geneve.ch
  Web: www.exit-geneve.ch

Founded 1982. Will find help for its own members who justifiably wish to die, according to Swiss law.

EXIT/Vereinigung für humanes Sterben (German-speaking)
Mühlezelgstrasse 45
Postfach 476
CH 8047 Zurich

Phone: +41 43-388-3838
Fax: +41 43-343-3839
Email: info@exit.ch
Web: www.exit.ch

Founded 1982. Will find help for its own members who justifiably wish to die under the provisions of the Swiss assisted suicide law. Had 58,000 members in 2005.

EX-International
C/o Peter Widmer
Postfach 605
CH 3000 Bern 9

Phone: 313-012157
Fax: 313-55561

Will help German-speaking people in Europe. (Note: The name 'EX-International' is short for EXIT and does not mean 'formerly' as in English.)

SUIZIDHILFE
Feldeggstrasse 65
CH 8008 Zurich

Email: info@suizidhilfe.ch

Will help with consultation only.

United States Of America

Compassion & Choices (C&C)
Two organizations under one board:

1. Compassion in Dying
6312 SW Capitol Hwy, Suite 415
Portland, OR 97201

Phone: 503-221-9556
  Fax: 503-228-9160
Email: info@compassionindying.org
  Web: www.compassionindying.org

2. End-of-Life Choices
PO Box 101810
Denver, CO 80250 USA

Phone: 1-900-247-7421
  Fax: 303-639-1224
Email: info@endoflifechoices.org
  Web: www.endoflifechoices.org

Formed in 2004 by an amalgamation of End-of-Life Choices (formerly Hemlock) and Compassion in Dying, C&C operates out of Denver, Colorado, and Portland, Oregon. The Denver office deals with membership, legislative and political advocacy, and local groups (chapters). Portland handles legal advocacy, services, public education, and fund-raising. Offices in both cities handle Client Services.

Compassion and Choices of Oregon (State)
PO Box 6404
Portland, OR 97228

Phone: 503-525-1956
   Fax: 503-228-9160
 Email: or@compassionindying.org
   Web: www.compassionindying.org/or

This group is the public steward of the Oregon Death With Dignity Act which permits physician-assisted suicide for a competent adult who is in advanced terminal illness. Residents of the state only (tax-payer or voter or home-owner or renter). In its first seven years it guided more than 180 dying Oregonians through the aid-in-dying process under the law.

Compassion and Choices of Washington (State)
PO Box 61369
Seattle, WA 98141

Phone: +206-256-1636
 Email: wa@compassionindying.org

Death With Dignity National Center
520 SW 6th Avenue, Suite 1030
Portland, OR 97204

Phone: 503-228-4415
 Email: info@deathwithdignity.org
   Web: www.deathwithdignity.org

DDNC works with leaders in other states considering Oregon-style laws, as legislatures, medical communities and the public come to understand the law's benefits as well as the choice, control and comfort that the law affords. It is the principal legal defender of the 1994 Oregon Death With Dignity Act before the courts, representing a doctor and a pharmacist against the repeated attempts by the US Attorney-General to repeal the law

Euthanasia Research & Guidance Organization (ERGO)
24829 Norris Lane
Junction City, OR 97448-9552

Phone: 541-998-1873
  Fax: 541-998-1873
Email: ergo@efn.org
  Web: www.finalexit.org

ERGO (founded 1993) specializes in informative literature about choices in dying. It updates and sells *'Final Exit'* amongst other books and pamphlets. Willing to talk by internet or telephone to persons or families about their right-to-die problems. Provides student literature and media briefings.

Final Exit Network
PO Box 965005
Marietta, GA 30066

Phone: 1-800-524-3948
Email: info@finalexitnetwork.org

Web: www.finalexitnetwork.org

Founded in 2004 by former Hemlock Society members who felt that the organization replacing it was insufficient and too restrictive about helping members to die. With its 'Exit Guides' across the country, the Network will help members who need not be diagnosed as terminal to achieve their own deaths. It also backs research into new methods of self-deliverance, promotes Advance Directives, and will advocate for people whose Advance Directives (Living wills etc.) are not being honored.

End-of-Life Choices Florida (State)
PO Box 121093
West Melbourne, FL 32912-1093

Phone: 800-849-9349 (M–F, 9AM–5PM Eastern)
Email: eolcfl@aol.com

Zimbabwe

Final Exit
PO Box MP 386
Mount Pleasant, Harare

Phone: +263-4-744258 or 308640
Email: frances@hms.co.zw

Founded in 1995, a small group of 617 members operating under difficult political circumstances, promoting Living Wills.

World Federation of Right-to-Die Societies

All but five of the 46 groups listed here are members of the World Federation of Right-to-Die Societies.

World Federation of Right-to-Die Societies
C/o NVVE
Postbus 75331
1070 AH Amsterdam
The Netherlands

Web: ww.worldrtd.net

Founded 1980. An umbrella group, it represents 38 organizations in 23 countries all working to ensure better choices at the end of life. It is now an NGO (Non-Governmental Organization) in the European Union. The Federation's 16th biennial conference is scheduled for September 7-10, 2006 in Toronto. Conference contact: info@dyingwithdignity.ca.

If you wish to add to, update, or correct any of the foregoing information for future editions, please immediately email Derek Humphry at ergo@efn.org

January 2006

Note: Closed in 2004 were: The Hemlock Society USA, Partnership for Caring USA, Last Acts Partnership USA, and Last Rights Publications, Canada.

CHAPTER 1

A jumble of assisted suicide laws.

Assisted suicide laws around the world are clear in some nations but unclear—if they exist at all—in others. Just because a country has not defined its criminal code on this specific action does not mean all assisters will go free. It is a complicated state of affairs. A great many people instinctively feel that suicide and assisted suicide are such individual acts of freedom that they assume there are no legal prohibitions. This fallacy has brought many people into trouble with the law. While suicide is no longer a crime—and where it is because of a failure to update the law it is not enforced—*assistance* remains a crime almost everywhere by some statute or other. I'll try to explain the hodge-podge.

For example, it is correct that *Sweden* has no law specifically proscribing assisted suicide. Instead the prosecutors might charge an assister with manslaughter—and do. In 1979 the Swedish right-to-die leader Berit Hedeby went to prison for a year for helping a man with MS to die. Neighbouring

Norway has criminal sanctions against assisted suicide by using the charge "accessory to murder". In cases where consent was given and the reasons compassionate, the courts pass lighter sentences. A recent law commission voted down de-criminalizing assisted suicide by a 5-2 vote.

A retired Norwegian physician, Christian Sandsdalen, was found guilty of wilful murder in 2000. He admitted giving an overdose of morphine to a woman chronically ill after 20 years with MS who begged for his help. It cost him his medical license but he was not sent to prison. He appealed the case right up to the Supreme Court and lost every time. Dr. Sandsdalen died at 82 and his funeral was packed with Norway's dignitaries, which is consistent with the support always given by intellectuals to euthanasia.

Finland has nothing in its criminal code about assisted suicide. Sometimes an assister will inform the law enforcement authorities of him or her of having aided someone in dying, and provided the action was justified, nothing more happens. Mostly it takes place among friends, who act discreetly. If Finnish doctors were known to practice assisted suicide or euthanasia, the situation might change, although there have been no known cases.

Germany has had no penalty for either suicide

or assisted suicide since 1751, although it rarely happens there partly due to the hangover taboo caused by the Nazi mass murders of the mentally ill and retarded, plus powerful, contemporary, church influences, and a law dating back to the Nazi era.

Direct killing by euthanasia is a crime, as one would expect after the barbarity of the Holocaust. In 2000 a German appeal court cleared a Swiss clergyman of assisted suicide because there was no such offence, but convicted him of bringing the drugs into the country. There was no imprisonment.

But the snag for German doctors who might be inclined to assist a justifiable suicide of a hopelessly ill person is that there is also a law that says it is a crime not to prevent a suicide if it is happening in your presence. (Presumably Hitler introduced this to take care of battlefield suicides.) While the banned procedure—voluntary euthanasia, or death by injection—is effectively instantly, assisted suicide—oral ingestion of lethal barbiturates—takes a few minutes at least, perhaps up to an hour. So German physicians generally avoid hastening death.

France does not have a specific law banning assisted suicide, but such a case could be prosecuted under 223-6 of the Penal Code for failure to assist a person in danger. Convictions are rare and punishments minor. France bans all publications that advise on suicide—*Final Exit* has been banned since 1991 but few nowadays take any notice of the order. Since 1995 there has been a fierce debate on the subject, which may end in law reform eventually. *Denmark* has no specific law banning assisted suicide. In Italy the action is legally forbidden. *Luxembourg* does not forbid assistance in suicide because suicide itself is not a crime. Nevertheless, under 410-1 of its Penal Code a person could be penalized for failing to assist a person in danger. In March 2003 legislation to permit euthanasia was lost in the Luxembourg Parliament by a single vote.

Tolerance for euthanasia appears in the strangest of places. For instance, in *Uruguay* it seems a person must appear in court, yet Article 27 of the Penal Code (effective 1934) says: "The judges are authorized to forego punishment of a person whose previous life has been honorable where he commits a homicide motivated by compassion, induced by repeated requests of the victim." So far as I can tell, there have been no judicial sentences for mercy killing in Uruguay.

In *England* and *Wales* there is a possibility of up to 14 years imprisonment for anybody assisting a suicide. Oddly, suicide itself is not a crime, having been decriminalized in 1961. Thus it is a crime to assist in a non-crime. In Britain, no case may be brought without the permission of the Director of Public Prosecutions in London, which rules out hasty, local police prosecutions. It has been a long, uphill fight for the British—there have been eight Bills or Amendments introduced into Parliament between 1936–2004, all trying to modify the law to allow careful, hastened death. None have so far succeeded, although Parliament seems now to be more receptive to inquiry and debate of the subject. As in France, there are laws banning a publication if it leads to a suicide or assisted suicide. But *Final Exit* can be seen in bookstores in both countries.

The law in *Canada* is almost the same as in England; indeed, a prosecution has recently (2002) been brought in B.C. against a grandmother, Evelyn Martens, for counselling and assisting the suicide of two dying people. Mrs. Martens was acquitted on all charges after a lengthy trial in 2004. One significant difference between English and Canadian law is that no case may be pursued by the police in England without the approval of the Director of Public Prosecutions in London. This clause keeps a brake on hasty police actions.

Assisted suicide is a crime in the Republic of *Ireland*. In 2003 police in Dublin began proceedings against an American Unitarian minister, George D. Exoo, for allegedly assisting in the suicide of a woman who had mental health problems. He responded that he had only been present to comfort the woman, and read a few prayers. The Rev. Exoo successfully fought off attempts by the Irish Government to extradite him to face charges in Dublin of assisting in suicide.

Consent Irrelevant

Suicide has never been illegal under *Scotland's* laws. There is no Scots authority of whether it is criminal to help another to commit suicide, and this has never been tested in court. The killing of another at his own request is murder, as the consent of the victim is irrelevant in such a case. A person who assists another to take their own life, whether by giving advice or by the provision of the means of committing suicide, might be criminally liable on a number of other grounds such as: recklessly endangering human life, culpable homicide (recklessly giving advice or providing the means, followed by the death of the victim), or wicked recklessness.

Hungary has one of the highest suicide rates in the world, caused mainly by the difficulties the mobile peasant population has had with adapting to city life. Assistance in suicide or attempted suicide is punishable by up to five years imprisonment. Euthanasia practiced by physicians was ruled as illegal by Hungary's Constitutional Court (April 2003), eliciting this stinging comment from the journal *Magyar Hirlap:* "Has this theoretically hugely respectable body failed even to recognize that we should make legal what has become practice in everyday life." The journal predicted that the ruling would put doctors under commercial pressure to keep patients alive artificially.

There was a heated dispute in Bulgaria in May of 2004 about the legalization of euthanasia. Its parliament spent a whole week arguing, ending up with the opponents getting a big victory by 93–5 for a complete ban.

Russia, too, has no tolerance of any form of assisted suicide, nor did it during the 60-year Soviet rule. The Russian legal system does not recognize the notion of 'mercy-killing.' Moreover, the 1993 law On Health Care of Russian Citizens strictly prohibits the practice of euthanasia. A ray of commonsense can be seen in *Estonia* (after getting its freedom from the Soviet bloc) where lawmakers say that as suicide is not punishable the assistance in suicide is also not punishable.

Progress In Four

The only four places that today openly and legally, authorize active assistance in dying of patients, are:

1. *Oregon* (since 1997, physician-assisted suicide only);
2. *Switzerland* (1941, physician and non-physician assisted suicide only);
3. *Belgium* (2002, permits 'euthanasia' but does not define the method;
4. *Netherlands* (voluntary euthanasia and physician-assisted suicide lawful since April 2002 but permitted by the courts since 1984).

Two doctors must be involved in Oregon, Belgium, and the Netherlands, plus a psychologist if there are doubts about the patient's competency. But that is not stipulated in Switzerland, although at least one doctor usually is because the right-to-die societies insist on medical certification of a hopeless or terminal condition before handing out the lethal drugs. Usually a non-doctor ends up handing the patient the lethal overdose to drink, and then reports the case to the local police.

The Netherlands permits voluntary euthanasia as well as physician-assisted suicide, while both Oregon and Switzerland bar death by injection.

Dutch law enforcement will crack down on any

non-physician assisted suicide they find, recently sentencing an elderly man to six months imprisonment for helping a sick, old woman to die.

Switzerland alone does not bar foreigners, but careful watch is kept that the reasons for assisting are altruistic, as the law requires. In fact, only one of the five groups in that country, DIGNITAS, chooses to assist visiting foreigners. When this willingness was published in newspapers worldwide, sick people from all over Europe, and occasionally America, started trekking to Switzerland to get a hastened death. DIGNITAS was overwhelmed. In 2001 the Swiss National Council confirmed the assisted suicide law but kept the prohibition of voluntary euthanasia. Then in early 2004 the Swiss Academy of Medical Sciences announced a complete U-turn in its attitude to assisted suicide, declaring that the country's doctors should in future provide the lethal drugs where circumstances justified it.

Belgian law speaks only of 'euthanasia' being available under certain conditions. 'Assisted suicide' appears to be a term that Belgians are not familiar with. It is left to negotiation between the doctor and patient as to whether death is by lethal injection or by prescribed overdose. The patient must be a resident of Belgium (pop. 10 million), though not necessarily a citizen. In its first full year of implementation, 203 people received euthanasia from a doctor.

Three right-to-die organizations in Switzerland help terminally ill people—their own members—to die by providing counseling and lethal drugs. Police are always informed. As we have said, only one group, DIGNITAS in Zurich, will accept foreigners who must be either terminal, or severely mentally ill, or clinically depressed beyond further treatment. (Note: Dutch euthanasia law has caveats permitting assisted suicide for the mentally ill in rare and incurable cases, provided the person is competent.)

The Oregon Death With Dignity Act came under heavy pressure from the US Federal government in 2001 when Attorney General John Ashcroft issued a directive essentially and immediately gutting the law. This brought on a public outcry that the Federal government was nullifying a law twice voted on by Oregon citizens. A disqualification of democracy! An interference with states' rights! Immediately the state of Oregon went to court (2002) to nullify the directive, won at the first stage, but the appeals continued into 2005 without resolution. Since 1980 right-to-die groups have tried to change the laws in Washington State, California, Michigan, Maine, Hawaii, and Vermont, so far without success. Thus in the USA, Oregon stands alone and under great pressure.

New Zealand forbids assistance under 179 of the New Zealand Crimes Act, 1961, but cases were rare and the penalties lenient. Then, out-of-the-blue in New Zealand in 2003 a writer, Lesley Martin, was charged with the attempted murder of her mother that she had described in a book. That same year the country's parliament voted 60-57 not to legalize a form of euthanasia similar to the Dutch model. Ms. Martin was found guilty and sentenced to 15 months imprisonment, of which she served half before being released, still unrepentent.

Similarly, *Colombia's* Constitutional Court in 1997 approved medical voluntary euthanasia but its parliament has never ratified it. So the ruling stays in limbo until a doctor challenges it. Assisted suicide remains a crime.

Japan has medical voluntary euthanasia approved by a high court in 1962 in the Yamagouchi case, but instances are extremely rare, seemingly because of complicated taboos on suicide, dying and death in that country, and a reluctance to accept the same individualism that Americans and Europeans enjoy. The Japan Society for Dying with Dignity is the largest right-to-die group in the world with more than 100,000 paid up members. Currently, the Society feels it wise to campaign only for passive euthanasia—good advance directives about terminal care, and no futile treatment. Voluntary euthanasia and assisted suicide are rarely talked about, which seems strange to Westerners who have heard so much about the culture of ritual suicide, hara kiri, in Japanese history. This is because, one Society official explained: "In Japan, everything is hierarchical, including academics, and government organization, and this makes it difficult for the medical staff and those who offer psychiatric care to join forces to treat the dying."

Another factor in Japan's backwardness on euthanasia is that some 80 percent of their people die in hospitals, compared to about 35 percent in the Netherlands, 35 percent in America, with as low as 25 percent in Oregon which has a physician-assisted suicide law. Euthanasia is essentially an in-home action.

Trouble In Australia

The right-to-die movement has been strong in *Australia* since the early 1970s, spurred by the vast distances in the outback country between patients and doctors. Families were obliged to care for their dying, experienced the many harrowing difficulties, and many became interested in euthanasia.

The *Northern Territory of Australia* actually had legal voluntary euthanasia and assisted suicide for seven months until the Federal Parliament stepped in and repealed the law in 1997. Only four people were able to use it, all helped to die by the undaunted Dr. Philip Nitschke, who now runs the progressive organization, Exit International. Other states have since attempted to change the law, most persistently South Australia, but so far unsuccessfully.

In a rare show of mercy and understanding, a judge in the Supreme Court of Victoria, Australia, in July 2003 sentenced a man to 18 months jail—but totally suspended the custody. Alex Maxwell had pleaded guilty to 'aiding and abetting' the suicide of his terminally ill wife, actions that the judge said were motivated by compassion, love, and humanity and thus did not deserve imprisonment. That was a trend in the right direction.

Yet it remains risky to help others to die in Australia. *The Bulletin,* an Australian news magazine, on 28 January 2004 reported these five cases then before the courts. Probably by the time you read this these cases will have been dealt with; I list them only as an example of what can be happening at one time:

• Stuart Godfrey, the son of former Tasmanian TV chef and author Elizabeth Godfrey, has been charged with aiding her suicide. That case is due to begin in the Tasmanian Supreme Court in February. He has pleaded not guilty.

- A Launceston woman, Catherine Anne Pryor, is facing charges of aiding the suicide of her father, 79.
- Fred Thompson, from NSW's central coast; he has admitted to police that he killed his wife, who suffered from multiple sclerosis. A decision by the NSW Director of Public Prosecutions is imminent on whether Thompson will be charged with murder.
- The infamous "21" friends of Queensland woman Nancy Crick, who were present when she committed suicide nearly two years ago. The Queensland DPP is still considering what, if any, charges those in attendance face.
- Sydney doctor Andrew Hollo, a former director of the NSW Voluntary Euthanasia Society, was charged last year with administering a potentially lethal dose of insulin to an elderly woman during a visit to her suburban Bellevue Hill home in October 2002. He is defending the charge. (28 Jan 04)

A further indication of the uphill struggle in Australia for freedom of choice in dying was the defeat in the South Australia Parliament in June of

2004 by 13–8 of a Dignity in Dying Bill. Democrat MP Sandra Kanck had tried before to get this passed. After this loss she said: "As the law stands doctors and loved ones are often left with the agonizing choice of secretly fulfilling the choices of the hopelessly ill and risking prison, or ignoring the individual's wish and condemning them to a degrading death. But one day this parliament will approve voluntary euthanasia." (The Australian, 6.3.04)

The strongest indication that the Western world is moving gradually to allow assisted suicide for the dying and the incurable rather than to permitting voluntary euthanasia comes from a huge survey that the Council of Europe did in 2002. It received answers from 34 Central Asian and European states, plus the USA and Russia. Not a few replied that such terms were nowhere to be seen in their laws so had difficulty answering.

Asked if legislation or rules made euthanasia possible, only one country (Netherlands) answered in the affirmative (Belgium had not yet passed its similar law) and 25 nations said definitely not. Asked if they had any professional codes of practice on assisted suicide, eight countries said that they did, while 21 said no.

Some of the other questions had revealing answers:

- Is the term 'assisted suicide' used in your country: Yes 18; No 5.
- Do criminal sanctions against assisted suicide exist: Yes 23; No 4.
- If so, have they ever been applied: Yes 6; No 6.

The Council of Europe, representing 45 nations, did not let the matter rest there. Its Social, Health and Family Affairs Committee approved a report, which called on European states to consider decriminalizing euthanasia. This was a massive step forward for the previously ignored right-to-die movement.

The commonsense of the Committee's approach is shown in the draft report by Swiss Rapporteur Dick Marty:

1. Nobody has the right to impose on the terminally ill and the dying the obligation to live out their life in unbearable suffering and anguish where they themselves have persistently expressed the wish to end it.

2. There is no implied obligation on any health worker to take part in an act of euthanasia, nor can such an act be interpreted as the expression of lesser consideration for human life.

3. Governments of Council of Europe member states are asked to collect and analyse empirical evidence about end-of-life decisions; to promote public discussion of such evidence; to promote

comparative analysis of such evidence in the framework of the Council of Europe; and, in the light of such evidence and public discussion, to consider whether enabling legislation authorising euthanasia should be envisaged.

Thus it was thrown back on individual governments whether to do anything progressive about euthanasia, or just ignore it, as most did.

Given this jumble of laws across the world, we need to look at the reasons why people are either fervently for acceptance of justifiable euthanasia, and why others are so nervous. It seems to me that the reluctance to change has more to do with attitudes to death rather than fears of that so-called 'slippery slope' towards forcible, governmental euthanasia.

CHAPTER 2

Beyond *Final Exit.*

If you could now look ahead in a crystal ball to 2050 or 2075, you would see a very different social attitude to dying and death. With the passing of those generations of us who came through the barbarous 20th century with its two world wars, atom bombs, genocides, environmental destruction, and polluting lifestyles, the new generations will be able to look with more commonsense and compassion on end-of-life decisions. All our present hang-ups, fears, and love of the status quo will be modified with the passage of time. Baby boomer generations are already making it obvious that they are either agnostics or 'Cafeteria Christians'—taking that part of a creed that they approve of, rejecting what they do not. Christianity and Judaism in the Western world will have to move with the times or fade into obscurity.

In the second half of this century, people will be able to 'off' themselves whenever they wish. The innate life-force will ensure that most people live out a decent span of existence, have small families, and contribute to the work force, while those whose health deteriorates, mentally or physically, will be able to purchase a suicide pill at a drug store and use it at their discretion, just like they purchase a gun now. By then we will have a more Oriental-like acceptance of the right to suicide.

Is the foregoing just speculative futurism? True, we are not ready for this now. We are too restricted by the left-over power of religion, the pseudo high morality of the media with its overpowering capabilities, and the 'head in the sand' attitudes of institutions such as the medical associations, academia, and political parties. 'Keep the status quo,' is their battle cry!

Better off dead?

In the brave, new world of the second half of this century, adults will have choices about their bodies that are not enjoyed currently. Only the Dutch and the Belgians have slipped the chains of old religious moralities, and have not only legalized (2002) voluntary euthanasia and physician-assisted suicide for the terminally or mentally ill ('unbearable suffering') but already started to debate the wisdom of elder suicide, those whose health is extremely poor but not terminal, and those who are old, frail, and tired of life.

On 14 December 2001, some 600 people gathered in a hall in Amsterdam to publicly debate elderly suicide. As far as I know there had never previously been a public meeting anywhere in the world with this particular agenda. Morality and philosophy played second place in the heated discussions to how a lethal pill could be developed scientifically, and how should it be marketed—on strict medical prescription or over-the-counter. It has been suggested that the government in the Netherlands run a controlled trial of a group of old people to test how many would make use of a peaceful exit.

The pressure to have such a public debate came from the huge membership of the Dutch Voluntary Euthanasia Society (NVVE). Of course, in the end the Dutch may not accept, or seriously delay, regulated elder suicide, but that will not stop it happening. The Dutch have sanctioned euthanasia by doctors in special circumstances since 1974, and it received Supreme Court approval in 1984. It is little known that the Dutch, in a very few, specialized cases, approve of the assisted suicide of a severely, incurably mentally ill person.

A retired Supreme Court president in the Netherlands, Judge Huib Drion, has been arguing since 1992 that those elderly who are 'tired of life' should have access to a lethal pill. He would set an age minimum at 75 with a requirement that immediate family be told plus a short waiting period. Already the pill—as yet non-existent—has been named after him, the "Drion Pill"—or in Dutch "Pil Van Drion". Without the benefit of a 'peaceful pill,' Judge Drion died naturally in May of 2004. Eyebrows were raised when the then Dutch Minister of Health, Els Borst, said in an interview that "very old people who are sick of life should be allowed to kill themselves." She did not retract.

The Dutch writer and cartoonist, Martin Toonder, 90 years old at the time, put the argument rather succinctly: "I am not afraid of death as it is the natural end of life. Dying is the ultimate detachment, it is a deed, a strictly personal act. That is why [Judge] Drion's plea to give old people the right to decide their moment of death for themselves by taking a pill, is not merely an opinion but an effort to liberate the mind. Freedom to decide that it has been enough, with all its consequences. So far, that freedom is non-existing . . . it deals with the very last decision man can take, the most personal, tender and intimate decision over his material life. Freedom to live means the right to die. We should grant that right to one another." (*Relevant* Magazine, vol. 29 no. 1, Jan. 2003)

"Lastwillpill"

Intending to make the elderly suicide pill better understood, in 2003 the Dutch right to die organization changed the name from the 'Drion Pill' to 'Lastwillpill'. The organization stated: "It has to be emphasized again that this development has to be completely and clearly separated from the euthanasia discussions. Euthanasia is meant to be a possible solution to a medical problem, while Lastwillpill belongs to the social domain as a possible solution of a social problem, both on the demand of the person involved only. (Rob Jonquiere, executive director of NVVE, in *World Right -To-Die Newsletter,* no. 43, April 2003).

To emphasize that there were fresh fields of ethics and medicine to conquer now that voluntary euthanasia and physician-assisted suicide were legalized, the Dutch Society for Voluntary Euthanasia (NVVE) changed its name to Right to Die-NL and resolved from now on to campaign for broader definitions of who could take advantage of the law. The Dutch High Court soon delivered them a set-back when it found that Dr. Peter Sutorious had acted illegally five years earlier in helping an 86-year-old man in poor health but not terminally ill to die with an overdose. "Being weary of life is not a justified cause for assistance in suicide, the court ruled." Dr. Sutorius had argued that the old man had lost 95 percent of his life's values: his mobility, his contacts, his will to live, the control over his bladder and bowel movements. "Death has forgotten me," the old man had said. Although found guilty, no punishment was given by the court to Dr. Sutorius. "Their verdict has created a new taboo," the doctor said. (*Relevant* magazine, vol. 29 no. 2, Apr. 2003)

In Australia, Dr. Philip Nitschke has defied the verbal censure of authorities all over the country by advertising and holding 'euthanasia clinics'. Since they started in 1999, more than 300 people have attended. The rampant Australian media loves to scandalize the clinics, thus they get plenty of publicity. According to Nitschke's newsletter, 'Deliverance', seven out of every ten people who attend the clinics later get what they want from their own physician. On principle, Nitschke does not himself administer euthanasia or assist in a suicide, but provides at the clinics information on how it is done, plus the where and when. While voluntary euthanasia was briefly legal in the Northern Territory of Australia, 1996–97, it was Nitschke who helped four people to die with a computer-controlled suicide machine. As with Kevorkian (except his last case), the person wishing to die was obliged to make the final move, in this case by striking a key. To Nitschke this method put the final responsibility on the patient; but he never ducked the help in the setting up.

Nitschke also says that of those people who seek drugs from their doctor, many report that there is "an unspoken understanding about the nature of their request ... the chance of receiving lethal medications from a medical practitioner varies with the nature and severity of the illness suffered. The more severely ill, the greater the likelihood that the patient will receive the substances they seek. (*Deliverance,* vol. 5, Winter 2001.)

"Although several options for those who are dying are canvassed in consultations, by far the commonest request is for some form of drug or substance that will guarantee a peaceful death. At present this is usually amylobarbitone (Neur-Amyl)." Those who cannot get drugs usually resort to guns or motor car exhausts, adds Nitschke.

The opponents of euthanasia have for years made the argument—specious for them—that if the dying and the incurable can have voluntary euthanasia, then why not everybody? Well, why not?

Nitschke argues precisely this. He says: "It's not uncommon that people get to a point in their adult life—possibly around 80—that rather than wait for something to go wrong, they feel in a very rational way that they've come to the point where their lives are best ended. It seems to me that that's a very considered decision." (Speech to the Hemlock

Society conference, San Diego, January 2003.)

A 79-year-old woman in West Australia, Lisette Nigot, took her life after attending one of Dr. Nitschke's clinics. Before she died she wrote to him: "After a long time when I was determined—but felt helpless and alone—to exercise control over the timing and manner of my death, it was good to know that, in fact, I was not alone. Your crusade to make help possible and legal for people who want freedom of choice in terminating their own life was an inspiration. I am sure you will succeed in spite of the narrow, bigoted and unfeeling attitude of the cowards who govern us. They have caused great distress and countered the wishes of a great majority."

Double Suicide

Although not dying at the time that they took their lives with an overdose, Sydney and Marjorie Croft, both 89 years old, who lived in Queensland, sent this last note to 'whom it may concern': "Please don't condemn us, or feel badly of us for what we have done. We have thought clearly of this for a long time, and it has taken a long time to get the drugs needed. We are in our late eighties, and ninety on the horizon. At this stage, would we be wrong to expect no deterioration in our health? More importantly, would our mental state be bright and alert? In 1974 we both lost our partners whom we loved dearly. For two and a half years Mary became a recluse with her grief and Syd became an alcoholic. We would not like to go through that trauma again. Hence we decided to go together. We have no children and no one to consider . . . please don't feel sad, or grieve for us, but feel glad in your heart as we do."

Established euthanasia societies are mostly uncomfortable with the idea of healthy people killing themselves. Generally this is political nervousness. For instance, it is argued by some that the Oregon Death With Dignity Act of 1994, allowing physician-assisted suicide in America for the first time, only passed because voluntary euthanasia was excluded and death could only come by the patient drinking a doctor-prescribed lethal dose. I do not think this argument is necessarily correct, but I am also sympathetic to the Oregon step-by-step approach towards eventual complete freedom of choice in dying.

A Hemlock Society USA policy statement puts its position thus: "Hemlock absolutely does not advocate suicide. Hemlock opposes ending one's own life for temporary, emotional reasons. Suicide is the ending of a life that could be rewarding and is never a good solution to an emotional problem. Hemlock does, however, believe that people with terminal or irreversible conditions that severely impair the quality of life should be able to end their suffering by hastening their death using gentle, quick and certain means." ('Frequently asked questions about the Hemlock Society," 2002)

The foregoing statement does not seem to me to rule out suicide for an elderly, ailing person in their right mind. In the USA, the elderly constitute only 12 percent of the population yet they account for 20 percent of all suicides. White males over the age of 85 are at the greatest risk of suicide. Very few are terminally ill, says the National Center for Health Statistics, which also reports that double suicides involving a partner or a spouse are most frequent among the aged. These type of statistics are surely telling us of the need to consider setting up responsible physician-assisted suicide for the elderly.

Those opposing the argument for allowing the elderly to get out while the going's good believe that the availability of a lethal pill will make murder easier. Particularly, they feel that granny will be pushed into the grave to get her estate quicker. These same arguments were made at the time the Oregon, Dutch and Belgian laws were being developed and voted upon. But it hasn't happened because well structured laws, with guidelines and penalties, are obeyed by the bulk of the populations.

Evil people will commit crimes anyway, and that is what custodial punishments are for. Must people like those mentioned in this book be deprived of a good death just because there exists homicidal enemies of society who are, thankfully, a minority? After all, only two percent of the 2.4 million Americans who die every year are suicides. The percentage does not change. That points to the natural life force to live as long as possible will be no weaker in years to come even when an exit pill is available.

Which brings us to the much more difficult question of the mental competency of those considering self-destruction. Even if you don't have all your marbles, does that necessarily deprive you of a choice in dying?

We can declare, in advance, that we may not want certain treatments if we become incompetent. So why can't we ask, in advance, for someone to provide us with a peaceful death if we become permanently incompetent?

CHAPTER 3

The enigma of depressive suicide.

When is a suicide not truly a suicide in the conventionally dreaded sense of the word? In my view, when a dying or incurably ill person accelerates the inevitable end of their life to avoid further suffering. A better name for this action seems to be 'self-deliverance' or 'rational suicide.' A raft of euphemisms have grown up around the subject: aid-in-dying, hastened dying, and assisted dying, to name but a few.

Many will disagree with my answer, yet there are a growing number of people in the western world who believe that self-deliverance from a terminal or incurable illness is not the same as 'suicide'. Undoubtedly, suicide is the correct legal term for self-destruction but for many people it carries ugly connotations of mental illness, depression, loneliness and desperation, while self-deliverance is seen as the action of a rational adult who has fought their illness, lost the struggle, and wants to check-out without more pain, distress, and the burdening of others.

Deeply religious people will of course feel that their Deity is master of their birth and death, and people have no right to interfere with His decisions. That is their right as freethinking people. All reasonable people realize that there will never be consensus on this issue.

The Netherlands, Switzerland, Oregon, and Belgium, have enacted laws permitting medically assisted dying for the terminally ill under certain tight guidelines.

The crux of the problem elsewhere is that, while suicide is no longer a crime (the surviving family used to be punished financially) assistance in suicide remains a crime everywhere except those places mentioned in the previous paragraph. But where does it stop? Who else might be deserving of an assisted death as well as the terminally ill?

For example, the suicide of Rosemary Toole, in Dublin, in January 2002, attracted attention because she was not dying and the police suspect that someone assisted her. Assisted suicide is a crime in Ireland.

Ms. Toole had told me the previous year that, at 49, she was tired of life and wanted out of it. She also told this to dozens of other people all over the world—via Internet and telephone. She asked people for help to kill herself, but not me because she knew I would not. I sold her the book and video of *Final Exit* as the least I could do for such an intelligent person. One could sense her desperation.

Myself—and I know others—tried to dissuade her, talking about better medications, more counseling, to hang on hoping for better times. We were all stalling, and declined to help her die. Then she told me that she felt better and would not go ahead. Yet she did kill herself, using a plastic bag filled with helium gas—a method quite commonly used nowadays by dying people.

Over the Internet, Ms. Toole had asked an American Unitarian Minister, the Rev. George D. Exoo, to be present at her death. He flew from his home in West Virginia to her home in Dublin at her expense. He has told newspapers that all he did was tell her how to do it, give spiritual guidance, and stand to one side as she inhaled the lethal gas. He does not think that what he did was a crime. For the occasion, Ms. Toole had dressed in a gold lamé gown, was well groomed, and smoked continuously. She had 4–5,000 pills, two EXIT bags, and four tanks of inert gas. Her 92-year-old father was in the house and seemed fully aware of what was happening.

Hers was a straightforward suicide. Obviously her deep depressive moods made her life not worth living. It is enormously sad that she would throw away her life, but, as she had made plain to dozens of listeners, that was her choice. Existence to her was unbearable. Like thousands of others, she would kill herself despite all our pleas not to. It was her life and her death.

Of course the question must be asked as to whether Exoo's presence in her home put a sort of pressure on her to actually do it? The rest of us were shielding our backs either on the telephone or Internet.

In the 25 years I have been involved with the choice in dying movement, I am frequently asked why don't we include severe, incurable, mental illness as a condition deserving the same quality of assisted suicide. For current political reasons I have usually avoided giving an honest answer. But cases like Rosemary Toole and many others make me stop and think: They're going to kill themselves anyway, so why not offer a modicum of decency in their act of self-determination instead of blowing their brains out all over the living room wall, jumping off a bridge, or spattering themselves on the sidewalk from a high-rise? It has happened that falling suicides have killed innocent people.

Journalists frequently call me to report that a mentally ill person has used *Final Exit* to kill themselves. What do I have to say? I decline to be apologetic. If the information in the book made their suicide less painful, less bloody, and less publicly embarrassing to their family, though I regret their passing, it was inevitable, and I can live with that. The real purpose of the book has been, in some cases, misused as so many things are.

It is curious that of the four people who founded the Hemlock Society in 1980, two committed suicide. Lawyer Richard S. Scott, a person with bipolar disorder, shot himself in 1991, while academic Ann Wickett, who had a borderline personality disorder, overdosed the following year. Gerald A Larue and myself of the original crew remain. I never knew that Scott was manic depressive until his best friend told me after his death. Because Wickett was my second wife I knew well of her mental troubles which had brought about our divorce two years earlier. But most other people thought she was a healthy person. In all other respects they were brilliant, good-looking, hardworking people.

It is fair to ask: did their latent tendency to suicide draw them towards helping to found the Hemlock Society? I don't know the answer.

Two Suicides

In my life I have helped two people commit suicide. People I loved. Both times it was a crime, although I have never been prosecuted. But let me explain the difference between the tragic Ms. Toole and the people I helped shorten their lives.

In 1975 my wife Jean was dying in England of metastasized breast cancer. Only 42, she had fought tenaciously against her disease, and the medical and nursing professions did everything within their power for her. She was not suicidal but a lover of life.

Yet out of the blue one day she asked me to help her kill herself when her illness got even worse. I agreed because I respected her intelligence, I had seen her awful suffering, and I knew in my heart that were I in the identical situation I would be making the same request.

Nine months later, with cancer throughout her body, she said she could not take any more. "Is this the day?" she asked, because our pact enshrined a joint agreement just in case the heavy pain medications were clouding her judgment.

She fixed 1PM for her departure. Sure enough, at that time she asked me for the lethal drugs which I had secured from a sympathetic physician.

She drank, murmured "Goodbye, my love", and died peacefully within the hour. (Her full story is told in my book *Jean's Way*) And this is my point, I was luckier than most people faced with this dilemma: Jean was perfectly rational throughout her illness so could make her own decision. Whereas the really hard cases are patients with dementia, mental illness, or Alzheimer's disease.

Eleven years later my father-in-law in Boston asked me to help him die. Arthur was 92, had advanced congestive heart failure and other health problems. We were good pals as well as relatives. I brought him the correct drugs; he drank them, and said, "Goodbye Derek", went into coma, and died within twenty minutes. It was what he wanted.

I wish I didn't have to have helped these two people die. Both times I broke the law but I am not a hardcore criminal. I have no regrets for what extremists call 'killing'. It was not killing; it was their hastened death by their choice.

They ought to have been able to ask a willing doctor for the 'Hemlock'—so to speak—and die according to their personal wishes. I was lucky that these two people whom I loved were rational and calm and knew exactly what they were doing in asking to die. They were also fortunate to have a helper in me.

But should people like Mrs. Toole be assisted in their suicide?

This is a conundrum society must face in this new century.

I believe the public in western society (and

dozens of opinion polls bear this out) is ready for lawful, medical assisted suicide for the terminally ill and chronically, physically ill, with appropriate guidelines. It has worked for many years in Switzerland and the Netherlands. It is the religious, medical, political and legal institutions which—head in sand—want to retain the *status quo*.

Assisted suicide for the mentally ill, or the permanently depressive personality like Rosemary Toole, poses far different ethical, medical, and legal problems, yet ones, which eventually we are going to have to address. Mental health problems are treatable by medications and counseling, but rarely curable. We know we are all going to die, and with terminal illness, we can see death coming, but do we know enough about the human mind to assist the mentally ill in their suicides?

Envy the Terminal

People with serious, protracted mental health problems have told me that they actually envy the terminally ill because at least they know the suffering is coming to an end before too long, while the suffering of the mentally ill continues as long as their body remains healthy—or they kill themselves.

Can someone deeply depressed ever be rational? Do they need to be if their decision was slow, thoughtful, planned, signaled to many others, and if they have exhausted all types of psychological help? I do not think we are yet ready for that step, although undoubtedly Exoo has set us an awesome question: Is the suffering of mental illness as worthy of help to escape from it as, say, the ravages of cancer? Possibly one has to have 'walked in their shoes' to really know who amongst us is the most deserving? Exoo would help almost anyone to die, so should there be any criteria to 'suicide on demand?' And who would set the standard?

Psychologist, suicide researcher and author David Lester says this:

"I would argue that each of us is responsible for deciding whether the quality of our own life is satisfactory. If we judge the quality to be unsatisfactory, then it is up to us, and us alone, to decide whether and how to change our existence." ("Fixin' To Die: A Compassionate Guide to Committing Suicide or Staying Alive." Baywood, NY, 2003)

While I know that society at large is ready for assisting the deaths of physically suffering people, we must first implement that resource, iron out any problems (as the Dutch have been doing meticulously for 25 years), and learn from experience. But we are not ready for legalizing help in dying for the mentally ill—that may come with social maturity in about another quarter of a century when we are better able to assess suicidal thoughts. While deliberate suicide stills tends to shock us, we should realize that only two percent of the 2.4 million Americans who die each year commit suicide.

And not all suicides get included in the national statistics. Many people manage to disguise their self-killing or it does not get noticed. Experts in the subject say the true figures are double, perhaps treble, the recorded numbers if the true facts were known. A small but fascinating illustration of this hidden truth is the horror a large and fashionable London hotel had in the 20th century of any of its dead guests ever being labeled as 'suicides.' The management had a private arrangement with the Metropolitan Police that nobody found dead in bed on its hallowed premises would ever be stamped 'suicide.' Heart failure or stroke was substituted.

This managerial attitude soon became known to the cognoscenti of the capital. Thus it was standard practice for anybody who wanted to kill themselves and not bring family disgrace—or lose insurances—to check into this hotel for their last supper.

CHAPTER 4

The denial of death syndrome.

A vast, mysterious chasm exits between those people who openly accept the principles of euthanasia and those who avoid committing themselves to it in any way. In Britain, with a population of 60 million and a euthanasia society formed as long ago as 1935, there are fewer than 20,000 paid-up supporters despite polls showing 80 percent support for law reform in the UK. In Canada and Australia, right-to-die societies count their memberships in the low thousands, even hundreds.

By contrast, non-English speaking countries such as Japan, the Netherlands, and Switzerland, each have right-to-die groups with around 100,000 members. In fact, only 38 out of 191 nations have any kind of choice in dying, proactive group. Membership of an advocacy group doesn't necessarily mirror adequately public sentiment in the Western world which seems to reflect close to two-thirds support.

Eventual death is something we must all face, but it does seem, on the face of it, that Anglo-Saxon-

Caucasian people are most in denial about this. Of course I take into account that many millions of people do not accept any form of euthanasia because of their deep religious beliefs. Nevertheless, millions of others who are not believers, avoid the topic like a plague. Not a few who feel their faith is in a Deity tolerant enough to encompass careful euthanasia, still do nothing about it.

It is also amusing how many people make the Freudian slip of saying, "If I die ..." instead of "When I die ..."

Various polls have put the acceptance of euthanasia in developed countries of the world at between 60 and 80 percent of their populations—a tremendous amount of believers but producing very few doers.

It is also noticeable, particularly in America, that famous people rarely lend their names to the progressive groups that energetically advocate lawful, medical, assisted suicide. For example, film stars Katharine Hepburn and George C. Scott spoke publicly about the justification, in certain cases, of assisted suicide, but when approached to lend the power of their names to an organization, either backed off or did not reply.

After starring in the film "Whose Life Is It Anyway?" actor Richard Dreyfuss briefly supported the California-based group, Americans Against Human Suffering, but let it trail off after a year. The rule of thumb in Hollywood from film agents to their stars is: "Stay away from controversy."

As long as a subject remains "controversial" a great many people in public life will instinctively avoid it. These are people who do not wish to discuss the significant social issues of the day, such as abortion, euthanasia, and the death penalty. As election results show, they will usually vote for the safety of the status quo rather than risk law reform. As any political campaign official will tell you, a "No" vote is much easier to obtain than an affirmative one. It took the all-powerful U.S. Supreme Court to legalize abortion in 1973 in order to bring some sort of calm to a splintered nation unable to decide for itself.

It has intrigued me for the past 25 years that a handful of physicians will openly work for euthanasia, even holding directorships of right-to-die societies, and giving media interviews, not caring a hoot for what others say. These rare people are secure in their work, firm in their principles, and know how to conduct themselves in public debate. Nonetheless, most physicians who work in support of euthanasia are in fact retired from active practice of their profession.

At the same time, most medical professionals keep their views on this sensitive subject to themselves. It is as if their careers would be blighted for life if they let it be known that they supported—if only theoretically—such a 'hot button' issue.

In Oregon, which has an assisted suicide law, I have come across numerous reasons for a doctor not wanting to carry out what in that state is a perfectly legal procedure, supported by the votes of 60 percent of the population. Even the normally timid Oregon legislature has added its blessing with a few extra alterations to the law just to suit the medical profession.

At the Bedside

During the six years 1998–2003 that the Oregon law has been implemented, the involved physician was present at the suicides of 70 of the 171 cases, despite the fact that all but eleven people died at home. In my opinion they should have been at the bedside of *all* the patients, giving reassurance, and on hand should something go wrong. Love him or dislike him, you have to admit that Dr. Kevorkian never left the side of the patient he was assisting to die.

It is not known how often all doctors refuse to help their patients die.

In the 'conscience clause' of the Oregon law all

medical professionals are entitled to withdraw. But the statistics which the law requires be published give us some idea: when asked by 70 qualified patients for a prescription for lethal drugs, 27 physicians over the three years agreed. In 39 cases the patient's own doctors refused. Other doctors were then found.

My own investigations into why some doctors decline reveal a multitude of reasons, such as:

1. It's against my ethical principles.
2. I don't want to become known as the local 'Dr. Death' like a Kevorkian.
3. Other doctors might not refer cases to me and my income will be reduced.
4. I didn't come into medicine to kill people.
5. My partners have threatened to close our joint practice if I do.
6. My grant from the government for research might be jeopardized.
7. I might be evicted from my offices if it became known.
8. I don't want my home and office picketed by pro-lifers calling me "murderer."
9. I don't know enough about the new law.
10. I'll write the lethal prescription but I won't be at the deathbed.

11. I'll write the second opinion on terminality but not the first.
12. I resent the way patients are demanding this new right to die.

Reminding these doctors that the names of all the parties involved must be kept confidential under the law seems not to sway those who are worried about getting either a certain reputation in their profession or publicity via protesters.

It was this 'head-in-sand' attitude of the medical profession that motivated Kervorkian to not only help people to die but make his notorious 'media circus' out of it so as to shock his profession into reconsideration of its attitude. Unfortunately, it did not work, and today Kevorkian languishes in prison.

While it cannot be disputed that all doctors, along with the public, are nowadays much more conscious of dying patients' cries for help—hospice enrolments are up and morphine is used more liberally—it remains doubtful if they are more sympathetic to legal assisted suicide or voluntary euthanasia. Has the juggernaut of the modern euthanasia movement, and Kevorkian's brief campaign, been a help or a hindrance in converting medical opinion? Just what did he achieve in his nine years in the public spotlight?

CHAPTER 5

Hemlock and Kevorkian.

When Gerald Larue and I entered the Los Angeles Press Club on 12 August 1980 to announce to the world the formation of the Hemlock Society, there were many doubters that we could last. After all, it was the only organization in America currently saying that assisted suicide for the dying should be seen as moral and made legal. Powerful New York groups such as 'Concern for Dying' and 'Society for the Right to Die' concerned themselves only with advance directives (Living Wills and such) and one of their leaders, hearing of the advent of Hemlock, opined that 'America was not ready for assisted suicide.' They made no secret of their fear that Hemlock's arrival would dilute the limited amount of fund raising that 'choice' organizations have.

President Reagan was just taking over the presidency with a right-wing agenda, and Jerry Falwell was in full song with his Moral Majority. America had, it seemed, lurched to the far right, with liberals like us pushed aside.

"They'll eat you alive," said one journalist to me.

"No," I replied. "Ours is a long-term struggle; Hemlock will still be around when Reagan and Falwell are gone."

Hemlock's shock appearance on the scene was on the evening news and in next day's newspapers internationally.

"Are you going to be in the Yellow Pages," a radio host asked sarcastically.

"Of course," I said.

When Hemlock was announced it had only one member. Within a year it had a paid membership of several thousand, and my records show membership was 12,927 in the far off days of 1984.

Twenty-odd years on, what has Hemlock achieved? Did Kevorkian's appearance on the scene ten years later help or hinder the campaign for legalization and the introduction of standards for a hastened, voluntary death? Some in the right-to-die movement blame him for muddying the waters with his seemingly indiscriminate euthanasia at the same time as they were trying to legalize a cautious, rule-bound way of death for a dying person close to the end. Others felt he helped by the enormous publicity he brought to the issue.

What is inescapable is that Kevorkian's actions set the agenda during the 1990s and he became the figurehead of the debate. But it is also inescapable that he was as much despised by some as he was admired by others.

Gaining the wide societal acceptance of the principles of lawful, medical, voluntary euthanasia and physician-assisted suicide was Hemlock's achievement. Before Hemlock's books and public relations campaigns, the subject—even in the two, much-older New York-based right to die organizations—was pretty well taboo.

Yet in its first ten years—and even today—the Hemlock Society's message appealed principally to the well-educated, white middle class. But not, incidentally, to minorities. African-Americans or Latinos were rarely seen at meetings. The fundamental reason why they stayed clear was almost certainly religious, secondly that this seemed to them to be an exclusively white, middle-class movement, and thirdly some feared it might be the start of a genocide of the poor and colored. In fact, Hemlock's membership was so extensively liberal as to be race-blind.

By 1992 Hemlock had 46,000+ members, had staged national and international conferences, published five books on the subject, and countless leaflets and fliers. Kevorkian's concurrent achievement, through massive media attention, was to introduce 'blue-collar workers' to the subject of euthanasia, although not always on his side of the argument. It was as though Hemlock, so to speak, was the tortoise and Kevorkian the hare in a race.

Over ten years Hemlock had paved the way for Dr. Jack Kevorkian's daring campaign of civil disobedience because by the time he started in 1990 prosecutors, judges, and juries in his three trials for assisted suicide already knew there was considerable public approval for his actions. Many were aware through Hemlock's publicity that in the Netherlands and Switzerland, the authorities already sanctioned hastened death. Were Americans that much different in their suffering and medical treatment?

Hemlock's biggest achievements have been in supplying the majority of the brainpower, labor, and finance for the six state initiative voting campaigns trying to legalize doctor-hastened death. Narrow defeats in Washington state (1991) and California (1992) were followed by two victories in Oregon (1994 and 1997), a heavy defeat in Michigan in 1998, and then a narrow defeat in Maine (2000). Hemlock and its supporters provided the bulk of the money, and the essential mailing lists of national supporters needed for these expensive campaigns.

Meanwhile, Kevorkian issued stinging public criticisms of all the attempts at law reform, describing them as too weak to be effective. As usual, the media played up his critical messages. A step-by-step approach to law reform is not in his psychological makeup. Kevorkian considers himself the messiah who will one day, single-handedly, achieve immediate social and medical revolution over doctors helping people to die. His condemnations were extremely damaging because they received huge media attention, leaving the average voter to puzzle: "I thought helping to die was what *he* was all about." Kevorkian called myself "another Hemlock hypocrite." My polite letters to him received no reply.

He publicly condemned (via a message specially brought out of prison by his lawyer) my issuance of the video version of *Final Exit* although he had not seen it. Sales of the video continued to soar, perhaps because people thought if *he* disliked it, then it must be good.

Hemlock was different from any of the 36 other right-to-die groups in the world in that it had always had a strong publishing arm. Between 1980–92 it placed its 'how-to' books on the open market, whereas other societies only dared publish privately. History books were joined in the Hemlock output by volumes on religion, ethics, and a bibliography. New books opened the door to radio and television shows, reaching millions, as well as providing continuous cash flow from sales. But today's Hemlock has dropped book publishing, switching primarily to politics. Hemlock's unceasing flow of quarterly newsletters kept its membership informed about all the trends in the movement, including Kevorkian's.

Somewhat to the confusion of the public, Hemlock and Kevorkian's campaigns ran side-by-side through the 1990s as each made their moves seeking the same result in different ways. By the Millennium, Hemlock was 20 years old and never stronger, while Kevorkian had lost his liberty. But Kevorkian had higher name recognition, nationally and internationally, and probably higher approval ratings because the simplified non-legal, non-political nature of his campaign resonated with the general public. He was easily understood by the average person whereas Hemlock sweated on the complex ethics and laws of assisted suicide.

Hemlock's Name in Question

Because of all the electoral activity in the states, new groups sprang up and went their separate ways from Hemlock, most notably Compassion in Dying. Their philosophy remained much the same—it was the strategy for achieving the goal that differed. This affected Hemlock's membership, which at one point dropped from 46,000 in 1992 to

18,000 members a few years later, although by 2003 it had risen again to 32,000. At one point there were eight right-to-die groups in America although this has shrunk back to four principal ones for 2005: ERGO, Final Exit Network, Compassion & Choices, and Death with Dignity National Center. (Some of these have sub-groups or chapters.)

Joining Hemlock was, for some people, purely a way of finding out how gracefully to kill themselves at the close of a terminal illness. For others it was more than that—to be part of a movement for a significant social change.

Thus successful publication of *Final Exit* in 1991 undoubtedly caused a lot of people to buy the book and not bother to join or rejoin Hemlock.

For instance, so impressed was she with this unique book that stage and screen actress Katharine Hepburn bought three copies of *Final Exit*, kept two at home, one on each night stand, and gave one to her friend, A Scott Berg. "Everyone should read it," Ms. Hepburn declared. (*Kate Remembered*, by A Scott Berg, Putnam, NY, 2003)

In the recent years, Hemlock—now wealthy from several large inheritances, and divided into two parts, one tax-deductible and one not—moved more deliberately into politics in an effort to get the assisted suicides laws modified to join Oregon, which stood alone among the 50 states. Already 25 state legislatures had rejected laws permitting assisted suicide, so it was an uphill battle. There was also a genuine fear that, with the Republicans in overall control of Congress and the White House, the Pain Relief Promotion Act (PRPA) would be revived. This Bill would give DEA agents the right to investigate physicians who were suspected of assisting suicides (of anybody) and make them vulnerable to up to 20 years imprisonment. Passage of this law would not only immediately neutralize Oregon's law but make similar hastened deaths a crime throughout America. It had failed in 2000 only because Congress was so wrapped up in impeaching President Clinton over the Monica Lewinsky affair that there was insufficient time left to get it through. Thank you, Monica!

Gallows Humor?

As it moved into the political minefield of 'choice' in America, Hemlock's many political advisors, strategists, and demographers complained that the name 'Hemlock' was a major handicap. Numerous focus groups said the same.

The hard core of Hemlock's nationwide membership did not want the name changed at any price. From its inception in 1980 the name

Hemlock stood out for many people as embodying the Socratic principles of discussion and debate over death. (Socrates was sentenced to death or exile by an Athenian court of judges; he argued that for him death was better than a lonely existence, barren of friends.) Politicians told Hemlock's leaders that the name had underlying connotations of poison and suicide which were a drag on the campaign. Some saw it as black or gallows humor.

Others argued that even if Hemlock changed its name to 'Grand Central Station' its opponents would know—and make sure the public knew—that the organization still stood for lawful, medical voluntary euthanasia and assisted suicide. But the board of directors struggled for a year to agree on a name, and then asked members to suggest a better one. About 400 names flowed in. After hours of agonizing debate the board still could not find a better name, suggesting to most people that 'Hemlock' was irreplaceable so why not leave it alone. All the most suitable names had already been taken by the other eight past or present right to die organizations in America. And Hemlock had huge name recognition which could not lightly be tossed away.

The argument for retention of the name was aptly put by a former director, William Batt, in an essay "Why Hemlock as a Name and Symbol' on their web site: "The choice of the Hemlock root as a symbol of our movement is quite apt for more than one reason. The first because it symbolizes the principle of personal choice central to Socrates' action. The second because Socrates faced choices unacceptable to him, much like terminally ill people today. The third because it focuses centrally on the place of self in society in a way that was vital to Socrates in his time as well as for people living today."

Hemlock also dropped its 20-year-old circle logo, a sprig of the weed hemlock bending in the wind, inset with the words 'Good Life, Good Death.' It was replaced by a bland line drawing of the rising or setting sun. The *Hemlock Quarterly* newsletter was first renamed *Timelines* and then *End of Life Choices* as Hemlock struggled to detach itself from its history as the largest, most outspoken, campaigner for the right to choose to die. It wanted to be in mainstream political America but with a tiny membership it did not pack much political clout.

Au Revoir Hemlock

As 2003 drew to a close, the leaders finally made up their minds, fixing on the name "End-of-Life Choices". Some members approved, others were disappointed. There was criticism that Hemlock had given up its decision-making to the many focus groups it consulted—in effect bringing strangers in off the street to form a decision which should have been voted on by members. Chairman Paul A. Spiers responded: "The new name is a more direct and accurate description of who we are and of the issues we support." One chapter leader complained that he could now be mistaken for a funeral director—offering burial, cremation, entombment, or burial at sea!

And instead of the old motto "Good Life, Good Death," the tag-line words of "Dignity, Compassion, Control" were substituted. (Please don't mention anything like dying or death!) Hemlock had just been scoffed at in a book by the historian Lisa Lieberman in her book *Leaving You*. "In America we prefer to address suicide indirectly," she wrote. "The titles of the Hemlock Society's two do-it-yourself books illustrate perfectly our culture's uneasiness with the very idea of self-destruction. *Let Me Die Before I Wake* equates death with sleep, phrasing the desire to commit suicide as a polite request, as if to suggest that the potential suicide will await permission before doing himself in … The best-selling *Final Exit*, subtitled *'The Practicalities of Self-Deliverance and Assisted Suicide'* is even more coy. Here, condensed into a single title, are two euphemisms for suicide—euthanasia as a 'final exit,' self-destruction as 'self-deliverance'—and a disclaimer confining the book's audience to people already on the brink of death." (*Leaving You, The Cultural Meaning of Suicide.* Ivan R. Dee, Chicago, 2003) Of course, as author of the aforementioned books I must take responsibility for the titles. They seemed to be right for the euthanasia climate at the time.

Undaunted by criticisms, Hemlock's board went ahead and changed its name to 'End-of-Life Choices.' It meticulously avoided words like 'euthanasia,' 'assisted suicide,' and self-deliverance in its new literature. Not a few members transferred their allegiance to ERGO (Euthanasia Research & Guidance Organization).

This was as far as the new management would go in its rewritten membership brochure: "We support laws that preserve our dignity when we have reached our end of life by empowering us to direct our own pain management and comfort care, *even to the point of hastening the end of life.*" (Emphasis added.)

It has always struck me as strange that Americans seem to be afraid of realistic words in connection with choices in dying. In the United Kingdom, the Voluntary Euthanasia Society of England and Wales has flourished under that name since 1935. All nine right-to-die societies in Australia and New Zealand have always called themselves 'Voluntary Euthanasia Society of ...'" It remains to be seen whether these euphemisms will win over support in America from significant politicians and be understood, and acted upon, by ordinary people.

Hardly had Hemlock changed its name to End-of-Life Choices when it the decided to merge with Compassion In Dying under a joint name and board to be known as 'Compassion & Choices'. Many staff were let go, including its principal public spokesperson, Faye Girsh, senior vice president and former executive director. Numerous of the original Hemlock hardcore people were offended at these changes and immediately started a new organization, the 'Final Exit Network'. The Network set its mission as solely to help suffering people, avoiding politics, legislation, and courts. It applauded those who worked for law reform but considered that as further legislation was many years away, what was immediately required was 'at the bedside' guidance by trained volunteers, as practiced in Switzerland.

Kevorkian's own book title was the ultimate euphemism, employing a word not known to the English language: *Prescription: Medicide* and subtitled *The Goodness of Planned Death*. Etymologists pointed out that if the word insecticide meant killing insects, and fratricide meant killing a brother, then 'medicide' had to mean killing doctors. Not what Kevorkian intended! Anyway, Kevorkian was now out of the public limelight in a Michigan prison —but he had left his mark.

CHAPTER 6

Requiem for Dr. Kevorkian.

Love him or loathe him, it is undeniable that Dr. Jack Kevorkian has engraved his name on the social and medical history of the western world. People in Australia or Germany knew him nearly as well as his fellow Americans. For the decade of the 1990s he was the most talked about, written on, and footnoted person in all contemporary discourses concerning the right to choose to die.

Now he is serving a lengthy prison sentence, his strident campaign for voluntary euthanasia over. But in that decade, through his actions, untold millions first became informed—and opinionated—about the taboo subject of euthanasia.

How he came to be so instantly famous without leaving the Detroit area of Michigan, which was his home, is an illustration of the power of the modern media which gorged on the story of the outspoken doctor and his highly controversial campaign for easeful death. From the first of his 130 or so—the precise number may never be known—assisted deaths, he was frequently the newspaper front page and television news lead item internationally.

Here was one person—an M.D. no less—who could feed the media's frenzy for a single individual through whom they could focus the enormously complex issue of euthanasia. Because as many people disliked Kevorkian on sight as revered him, the media did not have to worry about 'balance' in presenting his news. More excitingly, he had equipment the likes of which the world had never heard—a 'suicide machine.' With the issue grasping national attention, Kevorkian was heaven-sent for the media to improve their sales and ratings.

After 60 years of obscurity, the retired pathologist was the center of attention the instant he helped, in June, 1990, a woman with Alzheimer's Disease, Janet Adkins, to die with the use of his unique 'suicide machine' which he called a 'Mercitron.' Where other physicians maintain tight secrecy about their occasional administration of any form of euthanasia, Kevorkian trumpeted it, and even issued a video of Mrs. Adkins asking him for death.

He had put together from scrap piles, simple equipment with three bottles dangling from a bar. The first step was for Kevorkian to insert an intravenous needle into a vein in the arm of the patient. The needle was connected by tube to the first bottle containing a harmless saline solution which

Kevorkian started. The second bottle had a barbiturate sedative which the patient had the responsibility to switch if they still wanted death. The patient passed out. The third bottle, triggered automatically, contained muscle paralyzer, Succyochlorine, mixed with Potassium Chloride. Usually death came within 2–3 minutes.

An electric motor from a child's toy car drove the successive steps from one drug to another once the patient had herself or himself pressed the starting button. Death was almost instantaneous, although—as a lifelong student of the moment of death—Kevorkian meticulously checked this with a previously hooked-up heart monitor.

At first Kevorkian thought that the action of the patient in deciding the moment of death, plus instigating it by voluntarily pressing the button, might indemnify him in the eyes of the law. It would be them committing suicide with him a mere onlooker. But this excuse did not fly with prosecutors; after all, Kevorkian supplied the drugs and connected the person to them. He was the instrument through which his clientele achieved their ends, and that was sufficient to be a felony in prosecutorial eyes.

Kevorkian's first assisted death in 1990 caught Michigan prosecutors napping and helpless because, alone in all America, that state did not possess a law making assisted suicide a felony. In fact, in the 1920s the Michigan Supreme Court ruled that such action was not a felony in a case where one man gave a gun to another who shot himself with it. Kevorkian, a prodigious researcher in medical libraries in the field of dying and death, knew of this confused state of his state's law.

Three times he was brought to court on a variety of charges and three times he was acquitted. A local lawyer, Geoffrey Fieger, already brilliantly successful but unknown outside of Michigan, made a national name for himself with his feisty and shrewd defenses of Kevorkian.

But after some 130 assisted deaths, and now 72, the campaign began to take its toll on him, emotionally and physically. Doctors in the Netherlands, where euthanasia has been sanctioned for 25 years, attest to the strain of helping dozens of cases of euthanasia. Some retire from it to become 'consultants' to younger doctors. It seems that Kevorkian decided to wind up his campaign with one last, big, win-or-lose challenge to law enforcement authority. He knew he was playing for high stakes. His critics said he was deliberately martyring himself.

Thomas Youk, in the last stages of ALS, (in Europe known as motor neuron disease; in the USA as Lou Gehrig's Disease), contacted him for a hastened death. He agreed to Kevorkian's suggestion that this would be by euthanasia—direct injection of lethal drugs. Youk's wife and brother knew how much he was suffering and agreed that Kevorkian held the way to a compassionate death for their loved one. As he had in many cases of assisted suicide, Kevorkian video-taped his discussions with Youk, also the actual injection and the death scene.

After an autopsy, the local law enforcement received a death certificate stating that Youk's death was 'homicide'. They could have acted on that but, with the three past acquittals, plus public support for Kevorkian in mind, did nothing. Amazingly, the local prosecutor, David Gorcya, had won election to this office partly on a platform that it was no longer commonsense to harass Kevorkian!

Incensed at the inaction, Kevorkian took his video to the top rated television news program, 60 Minutes, which screened it shortly afterwards. In an interview with Mike Wallace accompanying the home-made video, Kevorkian issued a challenge: "Either they go or I go", apparently meaning that he would be acquitted of killing Youk or, if convicted, he would starve to death in prison. "I've got to force them to act, because if they don't that means they don't think it's a crime. Because they don't need anymore evidence do they. Do you have to dust for fingerprints on this?"

It was a challenge the hitherto reluctant prosecutor could not ignore. It was his constitutional duty to uphold the law as it is, not as some would like it to be. Within a few days Kevorkian was arraigned on murder charges as he insisted he should be. He was pleased. Then Kevorkian made a fateful decision which was part of his master plan to wind up his campaign with a flourish: he decided to defend himself. Being his own lawyer might give him the opportunity to go over the head of the judge, whose task it is to make sure the court follows the law, and appeal directly to the hearts of the jury on the grounds of compassion.

There is a saying that "An accused who defends himself has a fool for a lawyer."

Kevorkian well knew that if he failed to reach the hearts and minds of a jury who would acquit him, he would go to prison. But that did not daunt him, as his calm acceptance at sentencing and subsequent behavior in prison demonstrate. He did not carry out a previously-announced threat to starve himself to death once in prison, deciding instead to use appeal procedures to fight on through the courts

At the 11th hour before the trial opened, the

prosecutor dropped the charge of assisted suicide. This meant that the family could not be called in evidence to describe Youk's suffering and desire to be helped to die by Kevorkian. That left 1st degree and 2nd degree murder, and involuntary manslaughter as the charges.

What Kevorkian now ran up against was the inescapable fact that in Anglo-American law a person cannot *ask* to be killed. Euthanasia is homicide as the law now stands. So Kevorkian was thwarted by the judge's instruction that as a person cannot lawfully request to be killed, in a murder case he could not call the family members—whose testimony might bring sympathy from the jury.

This time Kevorkian was confronted by a jury which had little choice—given the video of the injection and the law as put to them by the judge—but to find him guilty of second degree murder. Nevertheless, it still baffled a large amount of public opinion—which doesn't think in legal terms—that helping a man pleading to die, in Youk's advanced terminal state, out of his misery could be 'murder' as it is usually known, which is robbing a person of a life they wished to continue. Hospice, which was providing care to Youk, had already notified the coroner's office of his imminent demise.

Kevorkian did not flinch as the Judge Jessica

Cooper not only admonished him—"Consider yourself stopped"—but handed down a sentence of 10–25 years imprisonment, the maximum sentence she could impose. He was given another six years for dispensing a Controlled Substance drug without a medical license. He was unable to ask for parole until six years had been served. In the first two years of his imprisonment, Kevorkian's lawyers three times asked for him to be released on bond pending the outcome of his appeal. This is a fairly normal procedure for non-violent prisoners. But Kevorkian had on previous court appearances given his word that he would not continue practicing assisted suicide, only to resume the moment he was available. This record of bad faith now kept him incarcerated.

Those who administer justice in Michigan seemed to have little sympathy with Kevorkian. His appeal, considered to have little chance of success, but to which he was automatically entitled, kept being delayed longer than that for other prisoners. Further, he was not allowed to be interviewed by journalists—print or television—presumably because the prison authorities did not want him publicizing his views on euthanasia. They made that rule apply to all Michigan prisoners. By contrast, the Oklahoma City bomber, Timothy McVeigh, while on death row was allowed to see journalists frequently despite the repulsiveness of his violent terrorist philosophy.

Disgusted with Hemlock

I met Kevorkian only once, in 1988, when he approached me as the then executive director of the Hemlock Society seeking my co-operation in opening a suicide clinic in Los Angeles. When I demurred on the grounds that we were in the middle of signature-gathering for an initiative campaign to change the California law on euthanasia, he stated: "You will get enormous publicity for your campaign if we open this clinic."

But I argued that Hemlock could not at one and the same time break the law and try to change it democratically. Kevorkian walked out in disgust and never spoke to me again. My letters to him were never answered.

At that point in time, Kevorkian, who had just lost his job as a pathologist to a Long Beach hospital, went home to Michigan to plan his solo campaign for voluntary euthanasia. By 1990 he was ready with his 'suicide machine' and sought publicity, soon getting attention from news magazines and major television talk shows.

Patients—or 'clients' one might call them— began to pour in. In his first year he helped only one person (Janet Adkins, with Alzheimer's Disease) to die, in the second two, and his big year was 1993 when he helped 12 people. The exact total is not known, but records indicate that at least 130 ended their lives with his assistance. Cancer was the main disease these people suffered from, and many more had ALS or MS. Curiously, considering its prevalence, Janet Adkins was the first and last person with Alzheimer's Kevorkian is known to have assisted in dying.

Kevorkian 'pushed the envelope' far beyond what the right to die societies in America were at the time working for—assistance in dying only for the advanced terminally ill. 'Dr. Death,' as the media dubbed him, helped people with painful terminal illnesses plus people with degenerative diseases whose life expectancy was unknown. In one case it appears he was persuaded by a woman in a wheelchair that she had multiple sclerosis whereas the autopsy later showed she did not, although that was her physician's diagnosis. In another case a woman was more mentally than physically ill.

Undoubtedly every person whom Kevorkian dispatched *wanted* to die. Nobody close to the deceased ever complained, although sometimes a member of a family who was at odds with the deceased while alive made a small fuss. Several accounts were written by the survivors and all spoke highly of Kevorkian's care and compassion for their departed kin.

The medical profession's dislike of Kevorkian stemmed not so much because he practiced fast euthanasia, but that he was not careful enough about medical evaluations involving a most drastic procedure from which there was no going back. He could not, they argued, know the patient properly—their financial and family circumstances, their diagnosis and prognosis—on the basis of arriving virtually one day in Michigan and dying the next. Kevorkian replied that he always studied the medical records in advance, discussed their illness with the patient and, if possible, their own physician. When they flew in to Detroit for the final exit, he would question them closely and record the conversations.

The medical professions' criticism of Kevorkian about not knowing his patients properly, and being a pathologist with no experience of general medicine, begs the question of what else were these patients to do because their own doctors had turned down their pleas for a mercy death?

They saw Kevorkian as their only hope of control and choice at their last gasp. In surveys and testimonies, many doctors have said that they had helped a patient die yet we know nothing about these patients and what, if any, safeguards were in place.

Before she died, Kevorkian's assistant for many years, Janet Good, told me that the waiting list for his services ran into the hundreds. He had turned down far more applications than the 130 he helped over eight years.

Many of these people turned to the right-to-die societies for advice and help. They got plenty of worthy advice but very little actual help, until later.

CHAPTER 7

As others see him.

Numerous academics have studied Kevorkian's behavior, the lives of his clients—mainly why slightly more women than men sought his services—his fearsome paintings, his composing of Bach-like music, and his Armenian heritage. But I'm going to leave the results of these investigations to them. (Mostly they are quoting themselves or each other.) Serious and long-term research on Kevorkian has yielded almost nothing of interest to the public or guidance in future legislation. Part of the reason for this failure is that some of the academics were instinctively hostile to Kevorkian and/or euthanasia before they started. Gone are the days when academia was not truly academia unless it was strictly neutral—the 'ivory tower.'

What is more important is how the rest of the world sees Kevorkian, for they are the medical professionals, voters, and lawmakers.

Satire and Sarcasm

As mentioned in the previous chapter, he has

long been the butt of many late night comedy show jokes, though few were clever enough to impress me, or even be remembered. They were mostly of this caliber: a comic referring to the new cinema release of "Lethal Weapon 3" quipped: "Dr. Kevorkian has been lined up for Lethal Weapon 4." Or in the major movie where Clint Eastwood catches a Mafia man about to jab a deadly syringe into his unconscious daughter lying in a hospital bed, and says in imitation of the Livingston adage: "Dr. Kevorkian, I presume?" Or skits about Dr. Death on the 'Mad TV' comedy show on cable television.

Andy Rooney, the long-time purveyor of droll comment at the end of the television news show "60 Minutes" interviewed Kevorkian in 1996, when there was this exchange. His approach to 'Dr. Death' seemed sympathetic.

Rooney: "I think the American public is puzzled by you. They don't know whether you're a medical philosopher or a nut. Which are you?"

Kevorkian: "Probably both. You might say I'm a philosophic nut, or a nutty philosopher. It doesn't matter. Words don't mean anything. If you dig into anybody's character you can find eccentricities you can characterize as nutty."

Sentencing him to 10 to 25 years in prison, Judge Jessica Cooper said: "This trial was not about the political and moral correctness of euthanasia. It was about you, sir. It was about lawlessness. You had the audacity to go on national television, show the world what you did and dare the legal system to stop you. Well, sir, consider yourself stopped."

Few have commented about Kevorkian in a more constructive way than Dr. George Annas, a bioethicicist at Boston University. An article by him that appeared in the *New England Journal of Medicine* (1993), and repeated in the Ohio Northern University Law Review (1994), warns the medical profession: "The real issues are related to medical practice, not the law, and the challenge Kevorkian presents to modern medicine is real. Physicians must respond by listening to dying patients, comforting them, providing them with a continuity of care and freedom from pain and suffering (even to the extent of prescribing drugs they might use to end their own lives), and bringing hospice into mainstream medicine."

"Dr. Jack Kevorkian is his own kind of ethicist, but if his bedside manner were not so startling, he would be seen as not far from the current ready-to-die mainstream," writes Nat Hentoff in the book, *Is There A Duty To Die? And Other Essays in Medical Ethics*, by John Hardwig et al. (Routledge NY 2000).

Who gets to make the final decision once the

patient has offered his or her life to Kevorkian? Carol Poenisch, whose mother Merian Fredericks was helped to die by Kevorkian, and has met him many times since, says under his rules "you can't make a generalization about who would get this and who wouldn't. Only Jack Kevorkian's gets to decide. He believes that it's case by case."

Brian Dickerson, a columnist for the *Detroit Free Press,* had this to say: "He was a polarizing force almost from the start. He was the anti-Christ for some, and a prophet, ahead of his time, for others."

Asked for his opinion of Kevorkian's promise from prison that he would not assist any more suicides, David Gorcyca, the Oakland County Prosecutor who put him behind bars, although not actually at the trial, declared: "The only thing which has ever stopped him from assisted suicide is jail."

As Human Being

"Thank God you are here,"—Loretta Peabody, the 39th person Kevorkian's helped to die. She had suffered from MS for 27 years.

His lawyer Geoffrey Fieger, asked if he and Kevorkian's were friends, responded: "Close friends. He doesn't like to express emotion, but I love the guy." On another occasion, Fieger stated: "What a goofball! The world will never know what

I have to put up with."

"Days Inn [motel] is too expensive"—Kevorkian.

"We love you, Jack"—Melody Youk, widow of the man whom Kevorkian was found guilty of murdering.

"… Kevorkian's flamboyant style—his outbursts and his antics—has fueled headlines, threatening to turn the whole matter into a serialized soap opera starring Jack Kevorkian." (Constance E. Putnam in her book *"Hospice or Hemlock, Searching for Heroic Compassion."* Praeger, 2002.)

As Physician

"I really think he needs to stop doing what he's doing. I think whatever good he's done in terms of raising public awareness of this issue is done. I think what he can do now is simply add to the polarization; he's going to be an example of the worst-case scenario of a maverick doctor acting on his own. And I think that needs to stop."—Dr. Timothy Quill, on PBS Frontline.

"Veterinary medicine," commented John Finn, medical director of the Hospice of South Eastern Michigan.

Cynthia Coffey, whose fiancé Jack Miller was the first man given assisted suicide by Kevorkian, said: "There's more doctor in Dr. K's little pinkie than all the doctors put together. He just came across as caring."

"I don't mean to put Kevorkian down. I'm just saying he's not the model. [Dr. Timothy] Quill is the model," said Faye Girsh, executive director of the Hemlock Society USA.

"Everything I see about Kevorkian puts in mind a person obsessed with death, a person who can't accept it and is trying to gain personal control and victory over it by saying, I'll control the timing of it."—Dr. Arthur Caplan, ethicist, on *Frontline*, 1996.

"Quill's the guy you want when you're dying," said George Annas. "Kevorkian's the one you want if you want to commit suicide."

Calling upon Kevorkian to stop helping people die, Dr. Quill said: "He doesn't have the right skills. This debate is not about suicide. It's about good end-of-life care."

"In five or ten years our society will realize his legacy and will realize the debt we owe this public eccentric. I only hope he lives long enough to receive the public accolades that he deserves."—Viewer's letter to Frontline.

At the end of their book *"The Suicide Machine"* editorial writers for the *Detroit Free Press* (a newspaper generally sympathetic to justifiable assisted suicide) said their book had "documented in exhaustive detail Dr. Kevorkian's reckless and self-aggrandizing behavior, his lack of standards, or accountability to anyone—including his clients and their families—and his penchant for making up things as he goes alone."

Dr. Marcia Angell, of the *New England Journal of Medicine,* commented: "The worst thing about Jack Kevorkian and his practice is that he's acting alone."

Dr. Richard B. Braunstein wrote to the *American Medical News:* "Kevorkian may not be the most appealing advocate for assisted suicide, but his was the only caring act rendered by any of Thomas Youk's caregivers. He helped Youk achieve peace and comfort." (In fact, Youk was getting excellent care from the Angela Hospice but that did not stop him from wanting a hastened death.)

A physician who supports assisted suicide, Dr. Ronald Cranford, commented: "I think Dr. Kevorkian is a nut. I think he's a complete kook.

"I think he's doing a great disservice to the euthanasia movement."

"It does disturb me that he [Kevorkian] has shown no inclination to expand his knowledge base and learn from others," writes Robert Kastenbaum, of Arizona State University, at Tempe, in the book *"Right to die versus sacredness of life"* (Baywood,

NY 2000). "A professional pathologist, he is not qualified as palliative care specialist, psychiatrist, psychologist, social worker, or nurse, to identify some of the types of expertise that could be called on when people are in situations desperate enough to make death seem the solution."

"Most physicians deal with life and death from the perspective of reason only, making science, based primarily on statistics from experimental data and case studies, the fundamental determination for life and death issues. Perhaps this is why Dr. Jack Kevorkian has evoked such a negative response from many persons who wish to take a serious and responsible look at the issue of right to die."—the Rev. Dr. David Richardson, in an essay "A Christian Theology of the Right to Die" in Robert C. Horn's book *"Whose Right?"* (DC Press, Sanford, Florida, 2001.)

"This [Dutch] tolerance of physician-assisted suicide stands in stark contrast to cultural attitudes prevalent in the United States, where right-to-die activist Jack Kevorkian's is serving a lengthy prison term for assisting in the deaths of mostly terminally ill patients."—from the introduction to *"Death and Dying: Opposing Viewpoints"* (Greenhaven Press, 2003)

As Martyr

The psychiatrist and author Thomas Szasz, who believes in a person's right to suicide, says of Kevorkian:

"Kevorkian remains important largely because many people in the media and in the country see him as a martyr to the cause of physician-assisted suicide: he helped suffering patients to end their lives. This is an utterly false image . . . Kevorkian urges us to delegate responsibility for suicide to physicians, promising benefits to those who 'need' it. However, since need is defined by the doctor, not the patient, the result is enhancing the prestige and power of physicians, and diminishing the autonomy of individuals, often at precisely that moment in their lives when that is all they have left." (*Fatal Freedom: The Ethics and Politics of Suicide*, 1999)

Kalman J. Kaplan, in the same book, reports in a chronology of Kevorkian public campaign: "December 31, 1997. Kevorkian's gives his 'martyr' speech in which he compares himself to other historical martyrs. He predicts that he will be convicted by the state and he announces his intentions to starve himself to death. This would implicate the state by assisting him in his own suicide."

"He seems to yearn for martyrdom," said the New York Times, (25 March 1999, p. A30.)

"I think he's been absolutely lawless, but I credit him with bringing to the forefront this very profound issue that faces society."—Wayne County prosecutor John O'Hair.

Asked where it stood on Kevorkian, the Hemlock Society replied: "Dr. Kevorkian was a pioneer who played a major role in bringing end-of-life issues to the attention of the American public, and demonstrating by his personal sacrifice the unfairness of current laws. Hemlock, however, stays within the law, and works through the democratic process to change the law where it does not provide for end-of-life choice. (F.A.Q. in End of Life Choices newsletter 2002)

As Humanitarian

Most people who admire Kevorkian see him as an outstanding humanitarian. This was confirmed in 2000 when Kevorkian—sitting in jail—was awarded half of the Gleitsman Foundation Citizen Activist Award of $100,000. Cautiously, the Foundation said that the prize was "encouragement for his activism but not an award for achievement." (The other half of the prize went to Bryan Stevenson, a lawyer who founded and leads the Equal Justice Initiative in Montgomery, Alabama.)

And in case any one thinks that jailing

Kevorkian is a drain on the state of Michigan's finances, that is not so. In accordance with that state's law, prisoners who have money must pay for their upkeep in prison. A court in 1999 ordered Kevorkian's to pay a lump sum of $28,039 from his personal bank account and $364.50 a month from his pension from the St. John Health System.

Disagreements

I have followed Kevorkian's actions since the mid 1980s, before he became famous, and have boxes full of newspaper clippings and television transcripts about him. But combing through these reveals that remarkably little was ever said about Kevorkian the man, the personality, the human being, whilst thousands of words were poured about the relative morality of his actions.

In a one-act dramatic play, *Jack Kevorkian vs. St. Peter*, the Hemlock Society's Faye Girsh, a forensic psychologist—speculates on how he might be judged at the gates of heaven. Should he be sent by St. Peter to Heaven or Hell?

Angel Gabrielle: *Please have a seat, Dr. Kevorkian. I have to tell you that I am pleased to be working with you. I have admired your career on Earth, although I admit I always thought you would not be a nice person. Sorry to tell you, but you seemed cold and even sadistic. You always seemed to be smiling too much when you talked about helping people to die. And you were such a loner.*

Dr. Kevorkian: *Well, I appreciate your candor, Angel. Or—what do I call you? Sounds like you've certainly made some judgments about me—like others I know. Of course, I see myself as a kind, compassionate person who has devoted his life to helping other people end their suffering. I do know that in many ways I am not like other people, but I know I am not an evil person.*

Kevorkian changed his mind about starving himself to death, instead deciding to sit it out in prison and keep appealing in the hope that the US Supreme Court saw things his way. But the court declined to hear his appeal, presumably because it could find no fault with his trial and was nervous about getting into the controversial moral issues of euthanasia.

Kevorkian's friends applied in 2004 to the Michigan Governor for clemency on the grounds of the unusual nature of the "murder," time served, and his health. Now 75, Kevorkian, with high blood pressure, could also appeal to the prison chiefs for a medical parole. Not that such would be automatic:

many long-term prisoners die of natural causes. Both applications were denied.

At the time of Kevorkian's third and last acquittal for assisted suicide, Dr. Quill put the doctors' dilemma very succinctly: "Well, we have a very funny situation about what a physician's responsibilities and intentions are when they are helping someone to die. Basically, you'll be allowed to do this if you really don't mean to do it, if it's unintentional. But you're not allowed to intentionally let someone die. That violates the arbitrary standard that's been set up.

"So, you can do it if you don't intend it, but if you intend it you can't do it." (Timothy Quill MD, PBS TV interview, 1998). With that deadly conundrum for doctors to ponder, the Kevorkian debate moved on.

Footnote: Dr. Kevorkian's rates an entry under 'personalities' in the Encyclopedia Britannica's Almanac for 2003, whereas Dr. Quill does not.

CHAPTER 8

The case for rational suicide.

The movement for pro-choice in dying is dedicated to the view that there are at least two forms of suicide. One is 'emotional suicide', or irrational self-murder in all of its complexities and sadness. Let me emphasize at once that ERGO's view of this tragic form of self-destruction is the same as that of the suicide intervention movement and the rest of society, which is to prevent it wherever possible. We do not encourage any form of suicide for mental health or emotional reasons. Nevertheless, life is a personal responsibility and some people are so tormented that they cannot bear to live. In such circumstances, understanding is called for. The reason that suicide is no longer a crime is that people can now seek mental health assistance and discuss it openly without fear of prosecution.

We say that there is a second form of suicide—justifiable suicide, which is rational and planned self-deliverance from a painful and hopeless disease which will shortly end in death anyway. I don't think the word 'suicide' sits too well in this context but we are stuck with it. I have struggled for twenty years to popularize the term 'self-deliverance' but it is an uphill battle because the news media is in love with the words 'assisted suicide' and 'suicide.' Also, we have to face the fact that the law calls all forms of self-destruction 'suicide.' Additionally, all medical journals today refer to 'assisted suicide' in their papers.

Let me point out here for those who might not know it that suicide is no longer a crime anywhere in the English-speaking world. (It used to be in many places, and was punishable by handing over all the dead person's money and goods to the government.) Attempted suicide, which hundreds of years ago in Europe was punishable by execution, is no longer a crime. Do not confuse this decriminalization with health laws where a person can in most states be forcibly placed in a psychiatric wing of a hospital for three days for evaluation if they are considered a danger to themselves and mentally ill.

But giving assistance in suicide remains a crime, except in the Netherlands and Belgium (also voluntary euthanasia, but both actions only by a doctor) in recent times under certain conditions, and it has never been a crime in Switzerland and Germany. The rest of the world punishes assistance in suicide even for the terminally ill, although the American State of Oregon in 1994 passed by citizens' ballot measure a limited physician-assisted suicide law. After court battles initiated by the pro-life movement, the Oregon law took effect at the beginning of 1998. After six years, a mere 171 had used the law out of all the state's deaths totaling 53,544 in the same period. Not exactly the stampede its critics were predicting! In 2000 and 2001 the US Congress was bent on invalidating the Oregon law by forbidding the use of Controlled Substances in physician-assisted suicide. That did not pass, largely because the State of Oregon, plus right-to-die groups, fought furiously to retain this unique law.

In May 2004 US Attorney General John Ashcroft was rebuffed in his appeal to the 9th Circuit Court of Appeal that the state of Oregon had no jurisdiction over the use of dangerous drugs in medical practice. Therefore, he claimed, they could not be used in physician-assisted suicide. This was his second defeat in the courts on this point. Whether the US Supreme Court will take the case seems doubtful, in which case Ashcroft may try in Congress to kill the Oregon law.

Even if a hopelessly ill person is requesting assistance in dying for the most compassionate reasons, and the helper is acting from the most noble of motives, any form of voluntary euthanasia (direct injection) remains a crime in the remainder

Anglo-American world. You cannot ask to be killed. Punishments range from fines to life in prison. It is this catch-all prohibition which ERGO and other right-to-die groups wish to change. In a caring society, under the rule of law, we claim that there must be exceptions for the dying.

Word Origins

The word 'euthanasia' comes from the Greek— eu, "good", and thanatos, "death". Literally, "good death". But the word 'euthanasia' has acquired a more complex meaning in modern times—it is generally taken nowadays to mean one taking direct action to help another achieve a good death at their continued request.

Suicide, self-deliverance, auto-euthanasia, aid-in-dying, assisted suicide, physician-assisted suicide—call it what you like—can be justified by the average supporter of the right to die movement for the following reasons:

1. Advanced terminal illness that is causing unbearable suffering—combined physical and psychic—to the individual despite good medical and palliative care. This is the most common reason to seek an early end. (And as Oregon research has shown, being a burden to others is an additional factor.)

2. Total loss of quality of life due to protracted, incurable medical conditions.

3. Grave physical handicap which is so restricting that the individual cannot, even after due consideration, counseling and re-training, tolerate such a limited existence. This is a fairly rare reason for suicide—most impaired people cope remarkably well with their afflictions—but there are some disabled who would, at a certain point, rather die.

What are the ethical parameters for euthanasia?

1. The person is a mature adult. This is essential. The exact age will depend on the individual but the person should not be a minor, who comes under quite different laws.

2. The person has clearly made a considered and informed decision. An individual has the ability nowadays to indicate this with a "Living Will" (which applies only to disconnection of life supports) and can also, in today's more open and tolerant climate about such actions, discuss the option of a hastened death with health professionals, family, lawyers, etc. But the person may not demand it.

3. The euthanasia has not been carried out at the first knowledge of a life-threatening illness, and

reasonable medical help has been sought to try to cure or at least slow down the disease. The pro-choice movement does not believe in giving up on life the minute a person is informed that of a terminal illness, a common misconception spread by our critics. Life is precious, you only pass this way once, and is worth a fight. It is when the fight is clearly hopeless and the agony—physical and mental—is unbearable that a final exit is an option.

4. The treating physician has been informed, asked to be involved, and the response taken into account. What the physician's response will be depends on the circumstances, of course, but we advise people that as rational suicide is not a crime, there is nothing a doctor can do about it. But it is best to inform the doctor and listen to response. For example, the patient might be mistaken—perhaps the diagnosis has been misheard or misunderstood. In the last century, patients raising this subject were usually met with a discreet silence, or meaningless remarks, but in this century's more accepting climate most physicians might discuss potential end of life actions, however cautiously. (In its Caring Friends program, Hemlock does not recommend discussing this wish for a hastened death

with a physician. One reason is that the doctor might eventually sign the death certificate as death from natural causes. Another is the fear of psychiatric hospitalization. Caring Friends' assumption is that non-medical methods will be used and no laws broken.)

5. The person has made a Will disposing of worldly possessions and money. This shows evidence of a tidy mind, an orderly life, and forethought—all something which is paramount to an acceptance of rational suicide.

6. The person has made plans to exit that do not involve others in criminal liability or leave them with guilt feelings. As I have mentioned earlier, assistance in suicide is a crime in most places, although the application of the law is growing more tolerant. Few cases actually come to court. But care must still be taken and discretion is the watchword.

7. The person leaves a note saying exactly why he or she is taking their life. This statement in writing obviates the chance of subsequent mis-understandings or blame. It also demonstrates that the departing person is taking full respon-sibility for the action. If the aim is to attempt to allow the death to be seen as 'natural' and not suicide, this note should be kept in a private,

secure place and only shown later if necessary.

Not Always Noticed

A great many cases of self-deliverance or assisted suicide, using drugs and/or a plastic bag, or inert gases, go undetected by doctors, especially now that autopsies are the exception rather than the rule (only 10 percent, and only when there is a mystery about the cause of death). Also, if a doctor asked for a death certificate knows that the patient was in an advanced state of terminal illness then not much fuss will be made over the precise cause of death.

Police, paramedics, medical examiners, and coroners put a low priority on investigation of suicide, particularly when evidence comes before them that the person was dying anyway.

Having considered the logic in favor of auto-euthanasia, the person should also contemplate the arguments against it:

First, should the person go instead into a hospice program and receive not only first-class pain management but also comfort care and personal attention? Hospices by and large do a great job with skill and love. The right-to-die move-ment supports their work. But not everyone wants a lingering death; not everyone wants that form of care. Today many terminally ill people take the marvelous benefits of home hospice programs and still accelerate the end when suffering becomes too much. A few hospice leaders claim that their care is so perfect that there is absolutely no need for anyone to consider euthanasia. They are wrong to claim perfection. Neither hospice nor euthanasia has the universal answer to all dying. For instance, 83 percent of the 129 people who have used the Oregon PAS law in it first five years were enrolled in hospice programs. Hospice may have eased their final weeks but it did not stop them asking for, and getting, physician-assisted suicide.

Fortunately most, but not all, terminal pain can today be controlled with the sophisticated use of drugs, but the point these leaders miss is that personal *quality of life* is vital to some people. If one's body has been so destroyed by disease that it is not worth living, then that is an intensely individual decision which should not be thwarted. In some cases of the final days in hospice care, when the pain is very serious, the patient is drugged into unconsciousness ('terminal sedation'). If that way is acceptable to the patient, fine. But some people do not wish their final days to be spent in that drugged limbo.

There ought not to be conflict between hospice and euthanasia—both are valid options in a caring society. Both are appropriate to different people with differing needs and values. Later in the 21st century, hospice will become a place where people go either for comfort care, terminal sedation, or for assisted suicide. It is the appropriate situation.

Religion

Another consideration is theological: does suffering ennoble? Is suffering, and relating to Jesus Christ's suffering on the cross, a part of preparation for meeting God? Are you merely a steward of your life, which is a gift from God, and which only He may take away. My response is this: if your answer to these questions is yes, God is my master, then you should not be involved in any form of euthanasia. It just does not fit.

There are millions of atheists and agnostics, as well as people of various religions, degrees of spiritual beliefs, and they all have rights to their choices in abortion and euthanasia, too. Many Christians who believe in euthanasia justify it by reasoning that the God whom they worship is loving and tolerant and would not wish to see them in agony. They do not see their God as being so vengeful as refusing them the Kingdom of Heaven if they accelerated the end of their life to avoid prolonged, unbearable suffering.

Another consideration must be that, by checking out before the Grim Reaper routinely calls, is one depriving oneself of a valuable period of quality life? Is that last period of love and companionship with family and friends worth hanging on for? Our critics heavily use the argument that this is so.

Not necessarily so! In my twenty-plus years in this movement, and being aware of many hundreds of self-deliverances, I can attest that even the most determined supporters of euthanasia hang on until the last minute—sometimes too long, and lose control. The wiser ones, too, gather with their families and friends to say good-byes; there are important reunions and often farewell parties. There is closure of wounds and familial gaps just the same as if the person was dying naturally—perhaps more so since the exact timing of the death is known.

Euthanasia supporters enjoy life and love living, and their respect for the sanctity of life is as strong as anybody's: *sanctity as distinct from sacredness.* Yet they are willing, if their dying is distressing to them, to forego a few weeks or a few days at the very end and expire at a time of their choice. They are not the types to worry what the neighbors will think.

Comfort of Knowledge

What people often do not realize is that, for many, just knowing how to kill themselves is itself of great comfort. It gives them the assurance to fight harder and therefore often extends lives just a bit longer. Many people have remarked to me that my book, *Final Exit* is the best insurance policy they've ever taken out. Once such people know how to make a certain and dignified self-deliverance, with loved ones supporting them, they will often renegotiate the timing of their death.

For example, a man in his 90s called to tell me his health was so bad he was ready to terminate his life. I advised him to read *Final Exit,* which he did and he called me back. He had managed to get hold of lethal drugs from a friendly doctor and so everything was in position.

"So what are you going to do now?" I asked him.

"Oh, I'm not ready to go yet," he replied. "I've got the means, so I can hold on a bit longer."

Now he had the knowledge, the drugs, and encouraged by the control and choice now in his grasp, he had negotiated new terms with himself concerning his fate. Surely, for those who want this way, this is commendable and is in fact an *extension* rather than a curtailment of life's span.

The Dutch have introduced, slowly over

20 years, laws permitting voluntary euthanasia and assisted suicide. The Belgians followed suit in 2002. The Swiss have always permitted assisted suicide—including non-physician assisted suicide—for altruistic reasons. The parliaments of Britain, Canada, and Australia, all rejected it in the 1990s. It seems strange, that Britain's parliament, regarded as the mother of democracy, has on eight occasions refused to pass a bill or an amendment reforming this type of law. Despite six attempts through state citizens' voting 'referendums' in America for limited physician-assisted suicide, only two have succeeded—both in Oregon. Nervous electors in California, Washington and Maine narrowly voted not to take a chance on euthanasia reform.

Nevertheless, thanks to the work in the last century of a forceful right-to-die movement, a hidden reality has emerged about terminal suffering, and before long the time will come for change. What are needed now are laws permitting voluntary euthanasia and physician-assisted suicide surrounded with a bodyguard of rules—but not so many that the patient cannot jump through all the hoops. With the inevitability of gradualness, that will happen. This is an idea whose time has come. Now we will look at where it might be going.

CHAPTER 9

Which way now?

Indubitably, the incoming Dr. Kevorkian stole the agenda from the mainstream choice in dying movement throughout the 1990s despite its being much older and experienced. The first euthanasia movement started in Britain in 1935, followed by the USA in 1938. More progressive than other right-to-die groups, the Hemlock Society, stood for the same basic principles as Kevorkian, had been started in 1980. Hemlock had been a darling of the media in the 1980s when 'assisted suicide' was freakish and new, but Kevorkian with his unique suicide machine was consistently even more exciting news in the next decade.

Between 1991 and 2000 the American movement fought six citizens' ballot initiatives at the polls—Washington, California, Oregon (2), Michigan, and Maine, in that order. No small achievement for such a small interest group. Four came close to winning (46–49 percent of the vote) but only Oregon won (51 and 60 percent). With the sincerity and professionalism of these attempts democratically to reform the law, Hemlock, and companion groups such as Oregon Right to Die, still held the high moral ground throughout. At first these initiative campaigns drew enormous media attention, but as, one by one, they narrowly failed, media interested dwindled. Meanwhile, Kevorkian constantly snatched the headlines and the public's attention. The general public began to equate the whole death with dignity discussion chiefly with Kevorkian—who had no interest in law reform—and their ownership of the 'high ground' was not much use politically to the pro-choice groups, whose leaders considered him an unwanted distraction and a poor example.

For example, Kevorkian's—representing only himself—was twice asked to address the National Press Club, in Washington DC, but no spokesperson for the mainstream right-to-die groups, supported by millions, was ever invited to offer an alternative strategy.

Scarcity of coalitions

During all the political campaigns, professionals urged the right-to-die groups to form coalitions in order to widen their public support. You couldn't hope to win without that cooperation, went the advice. But it was not that easy. First, most organizations are short of quality volunteers and have few paid staff. They can't spare the time to work on someone else's project, nor even attend working committees.

Secondly, groups like NARAL, ACLU, NOW, and Amnesty International already face enough criticism and protest from the religious right without the intensely controversial issue of euthanasia being added to their agenda. Granted, the ACLU has always been supportive of the right-to-die movement on a case-by-case basis, and helped defend the Oregon law in the courts.

Fourthly, civil liberty groups fear losing their donation base to other liberal groups as each learns who are each others biggest contributors. (The same goes for right wing and anti-choice groups.)

In California and Washington, much—too much—was expected from the gay community at the height of the AIDS epidemic in the 1990s.

Assisted suicides between victims—at great legal risk, and often botched—was fairly common. For instance, Americans Against Human Suffering, as part of its 1992 ballot initiative sought the backing of the gay community in San Francisco, which was extremely well organized. No assistance came. The best and the brightest in gay society were too busy raising money for AIDS hospices, and of course from their point of view this was the priority.

Looking to the churches was equally frustrating. The Roman Catholic hierarchy was, of course, strongly opposed, while the Episcopalians were divided. Lutherans and Baptists were opposed, while Methodists on the West Coast leaned tentatively towards support. Only the Unitarian Universalist Association gave its complete backing, but that is one of the smallest churches in America.

Sociologist Joe Bandy, of Bowdoin University, has argued that "without coalitions with church groups, as other progressive social causes have done in the past (Black civil rights as the outstanding example), the movement for choice in dying will be severely handicapped." (Talk to the 2000 world euthanasia conference in Boston.) Good advice, but how is this going to happen soon, if at all? There is no more divisive issue between people of intelligence than euthanasia—more divisive than abortion because it affects everybody whereas abortion touches only a few. With abortions we are arguing about other peoples' rights and needs; with euthanasia it is about our individual rights and ethics.

Funding
All the socially progressive nonprofit groups complain of under-funding. That is because they

are young and unlikely to have any regular source of income, such as endowments, currently depending entirely on the whims of their donation base in response to mass mailings. Plus, they naturally always want to be doing better work than they are currently.

In the initiative campaigns in California and Michigan, there was a severe shortage of funds. But that was largely due to the widely held view that these two campaigns were doomed to lose anyway. However, in Washington State there was no shortage of money, but it was spent too soon and unwisely. Oregon, which had to fight two bitter citizens' ballot campaigns before the Death With Dignity Act became law, and although outspent by the opposition, was fairly well funded, and spent its cash shrewdly. Significantly, Oregon was the first time some multi-millionaires like George Soros came forward with massive individual contributions of six figures. In the last campaign in Maine in 2000, there was no lack of pro-choice funds. In all these campaigns, the Roman Catholic Church, national and local, was the chief financier in opposition to euthanasia, whilst the Hemlock Society, nationally and locally, was the main backer on the pro side. (The Hemlock Society had 32,000 members; the Roman Catholic Church in America had

61 million. The National Right to Life Committee boasts 15 million members.)

In the final testing of a citizens' vote on an issue involving moral behavior, it is not the money that counts— though it helps enormously. The true test is whether a majority of the voters are sufficiently convinced to take the plunge on euthanasia law reform. In all five campaigns, voter support was always highest a few months prior to Election Day. But as the opposing groups chiseled away at the law with expensive television advertisements, repetitively insisting that it was weak, poorly drafted, and dangerous to old and disabled people, voter confidence always faded.

The Enigma of Oregon

Why has Oregon, alone of all the 50 states, not only voted twice (51 percent in 1994, then confirmed by 60 percent in 1997) to have a law allowing medically-assisted suicide for its dying residents? Even a hostile legislature, gasping to overturn this, to them, awful law, was afraid to defy the public over this. Fearing voter backlash, legislators ended up making minor alterations, mostly to please the hospitals. For several years, opponents in the US Congress have been maneuvering to find ways to kill off the Oregon law but had not succeeded as of

July 2004. And as was reported earlier, two senior courts on the West coast rejected the US attorney-general's attempts to quash the Oregon law. Now in its seventh year, without problems and gaining stature, Oregon's law was setting an example which other states could emulate.

Why Oregon? Having been a resident of the state for the last 13 years, and founder of the state's Hemlock Chapter in 1987, I am expected to know the answer. I'll try. As might be expected, Oregon's unique position in pro-choice issues is a combination of factors, some inherent, some planned, plus a few bits of luck in timing.

Populated to quite a large degree by descendents of the original 'Oregon Trail' pioneers of the 19th century, Oregon people are consistently liberal when to comes to causes such as animal rights, gay rights, freedom of speech, and abortion rights. Not that people in neighboring California and Washington aren't also liberal (four million in California voted pro-choice in dying in 1992), but in Oregon freedom of thought is more deeply entrenched. For example, Oregon pioneered the citizen initiative voting system early in the 20th century, was the first with planning laws, and can and bottle recycling requirements.

A state of only 3–4 million people, surveys

repeatedly show that fewer attend church, on average, than any other US state. It is not necessarily that they are more ungodly, but they resent authority, preferring to fish on Sunday mornings. The Oregon state motto, translated from the Latin, means: "She flies with her own wings."

The road to pro-choice in dying in Oregon began in 1993 when a group of Hemlock members in Portland watched closely the defeats in Washington and California, the states above and below them geographically. A Political Action Committee (PAC) was formed which brainstormed for the answer as to why voter support always slipped away just before polling day. The problems of shortage of money, and tactless use of it, were soon resolved. There must be something deeper.

The brains trust, comprising Eli Stutsman, Barbara Coombs Lee, Jeff Sugarman, Peter Goodwin and the late Elvin Sinnard, concluded that they might win if they eliminated from their proposed law the legalization of voluntary euthanasia (lethal injection by doctor). A cautious law permitting only physician-assisted suicide was framed. Euthanasia was specifically prohibited. Goodwin, a physician, argued that doctors dreaded putting a needle containing deadly drugs into a patient's arm. It was too similar to murder. But they were not so sensitive about prescribing a lethal cocktail, letting the patient fill it, and—if still so minded—drink it and die. 'Assisting a suicide' (in justifiable circumstances) was more acceptable to them than 'killing'. Sugarman, a political professional, felt that putting the responsibility for causing death directly upon the patient, and only indirectly on the doctor, would stem the catastrophic late loss of votes previously experienced.

At one swipe, the level of assistance in death, which Hemlock had been advocating for 13 years, was halved. I disagreed with this severance, but the PAC members argued that, after two previous defeats at the polls, it couldn't afford another near miss, and the movement needed a change of strategy from voluntary euthanasia and assisted suicide to one of step-by-step. The voters might stick with this.

My disagreement was based on several things:

(a) patients who could not swallow a liquid remained unhelped, and often it they who most needed assistance, particularly after throat and stomach cancer;

(b) it was a dishonest step back from years of promises by Hemlock to its members;

(c) the public was not interested in the medical and ethical niceties of the law; what it wanted was gentle, easy death similar to the way it appeared to them that Dr. Kevorkian did things;

(d) The anti-choice forces would fight us just as hard even if the proposed law were watered down.

But it was the brain trust's show and they went ahead, got the necessary signatures on a petition, and polling of the Oregon electorate was fixed for 4 November 1994. This time there were almost no public meetings and the 'Yes' campaign was confined to newspaper coverage, and in the last week a blast of television advertising. (I confined myself to raising money for the campaign.) Oregon's newspapers took sides editorially on the issue—for instance, the biggest, *The Oregonian*, was campaigning furiously for a 'No' vote, whilst the 2nd largest, *The Register-Guard*, of Eugene, was calmly advocating a 'Yes.'

The Death With Dignity Act became law in 1994, by 51-49 percent, but was held up for the next three years by a series of lawsuits brought by the pro-life side. They came to naught, except securing time for maneuvering behind the political scenes. Some five bills were introduced into the legislature which would have nullified or made unworkable the new law. Democrats argued that it would be sufficient to tidy up any flaws and leave it alone. The Republicans, in the majority, refused to touch the law, desiring to send it back to the electorate in its present state. This they did. It was the first time in 86 years that the legislature had the cheek to ask the voters to think again on exactly the same law. It was a huge mistake.

A furious campaign for repeal of the law continued throughout 1998. The churches, particularly Roman Catholics ones, poured most of the $4,077,882 which went into the "Yes" on repeal campaign. (Compared to $966,000 by the campaign to keep the law.) But this time the pro-choice side had two things going for it:

1. It is easier to get a 'No' vote than a 'Yes' one.
2. A considerable section of the electorate was angry at being told to vote a second time, and protested this by voting 'No'.

By the end of polling day, the repeal of the law had been defeated by 60-40 percent. The right wing was dumb-founded at their crushing loss. From a slender victory in 1994, the pro-choice side had been handed a substantial mandate by the public. The law took effect in November 1997, but for all practical purposes, including statistics, it began the first day of 1998. (For figures on the use dying people made of the law, see appendix C.)

After an unsuccessful attempt to get the Justice Department to intervene against it through Attorney General Janet Reno, over the next three years the battle to kill the Oregon law shifted to the US

Congress. Luckily for its supporters, Congress was trying to impeach President Clinton for the Monica Lewinsky affair and other things. This greatly added to their business agenda and the Pain Relief Promotion Act, intended to prevent any doctor in America from prescribing Controlled Substances (including, of course, barbiturates) was stalled. It easily passed the House of Representatives but the Senate put it at the bottom of their agenda. By the time of the General Election in 2000, narrowly won by George W. Bush, it was still loitering somewhere in the Senate cubbyholes.

Why Not Maine?

Defiantly, in the middle of this kafuffle, the Hemlock Society chapter in Maine decided to try to their luck with a voter initiative campaign since the legislature had repeatedly thrown out a law similar to Oregon's muted one. Maine is similar to Oregon not only in size but also with the same tendency to support liberal causes, except that 30 percent of its citizens are French-Catholics. If there could be two states with roughly the same law, the reasoning went, the opponents would find it harder to challenge. Dr. Kevorkian was locked away in prison so could not butt in on the proceedings. Now the opposition could no longer claim that he might set up a clinic in Maine as they had pointed out in previous elections, hoping to scare the voters.

The 'Yes' campaign received massive support from the national Hemlock Society, its members, and its chapters. The 'No' side were well organized and well financed. Opinion polls pointed to a comfortable victory for pro-choice. Yet in the end they were wrong. At the last minute, because of deceptive TV advertisements, the Maine voter support slipped away and the assisted suicide law was rejected 49–51 percent. A narrow loss, but a loss just the same.

What went wrong was that the once highly controversial issue of assisted suicide had faded in importance in the public conscience. Maine's newspapers rarely reported the campaign except when opinion polls were issued. Pro-choice leaders holding press conferences found the media uninformed and disinterested. The churches kept a low profile and nobody cared—as they had done in Oregon—that religious organizations were calling the shots behind the scenes. What seemed most to contribute to Hemlock's defeat was that Maine's doctors, nurses, and hospices, organized groups to fight the law reform. Quite naturally, the ordinary voter would be thinking that if his health professionals were against the new law, then it was safer to side with them.

In Maine there was no public fight, and name-calling, as there had been in Oregon. So the old bogy of voters voting "No" for the safety of the status quo prevailed. By now, after five similar campaigns, the anti-choice side knew exactly how to pitch its television advertising: hammer away that the law is 'poorly drafted and dangerous.' Right-to-die leaders keen for law reform felt 'dead in the water' after the Maine fiasco into which so much effort and money had been poured. What should be done next?

CHAPTER 10

Pendulum.

All things come to pass with patience, money and time, says the 17th century proverb. And so it will be with choice in dying, except that it will also need what the proverb omits: *effort*. Not 'big time' effort such as a $10 million advertising campaign or Billy Graham-type evangelizing tour, but the solid type of work that quietly, steadily, over years convinces people that this is laudable reform which they can support for themselves and others.

It is well proven through the voting system in America that 50 percent of the public supports lawful, medical assisted dying. Another 20 percent are not too sure. (They are the floating vote that says "Yes" in advance but retreats when faced with a final decision in the polling booth.) Support is similar in most other developed countries, with only the Netherlands and Belgium achieving any progress so far.

One cannot compare the manner of social progress in European countries (one government each) with that of the USA (50 state governments),

Australia (6 Plus 2 Territories). Canada has a Federal penal code. Not only are these multi-ethnic and multi-cultural nations but great power lies within their states, making something as divisive ethically as euthanasia, which needs a national policy, extremely difficult on which to gain consensus of a majority needed to change law.

Compassion

Since Ralph Mero started 'Compassion in Dying' in Seattle in 1993, there has been a growing realization that more can be done in a practical way for those who want assisted suicide than was originally thought by the early leaders, who feared legal repercussions. Mero demonstrated that there was a significant level of worthwhile help that could be given without breaking the law. Times had changed; the taboo concerning assisted death had been broken down in the 1980s. From 1990 onwards there was Dr. Kevorkian and the national best-selling book *Final Exit*, plus almost yearly election campaigns on the issue.

When it received a cry for help from a patient, Compassion in Dying checked out the situation with a home visit by an experienced counselor. More often than not the problem was the hesitation of the family doctor, who had never met such a request before and did not know how to deal with it ethically, legally, or medically. In a good many cases a call from one of Compassion's medical team to discuss the problems with the family doctor got over the difficulties. Just as lawyers listen to lawyers, doctors listen to doctors—a feature of professional pride. If the family doctor still declined, another doctor who was willing to cooperate was found.

Caring Friends Starts

Compassion's work was confined to Washington State for a few years because, after the electoral victories in Oregon, almost the whole movement—including me—optimistically thought that there would now be a domino effect for law reform across most states except the South. This, as has been said, did not happen. Therefore, as the 20th century drew to a close, Hemlock proceeded to form an outreach arm called 'Caring Friends', run out of its headquarters in Denver, but available to every member with a documented terminal or hopeless illness who was eligible—at no cost.

When *Final Exit* appeared in 1991, Hemlock recommended it to people whose illnesses had progressed to the point where they were considering a hastened death and wanted help. It became clear, in 1998, that reading a book to achieve a peaceful death was not enough for some people. A major donor to Hemlock ended her suffering with lung cancer by shooting herself; she was alone and her body was found by a young woman going to work.

Even with the good advice in the book, many people at the end of their lives were too debilitated, too frightened, too sick, or too alone to use a book to help them to die. Also, they were increasingly unable to obtain the necessary medications as governments tightened their holds on dangerous drugs. What was needed was a program where trained Hemlock members could work with another member who, because of the nature of their underlying illness, were considering hastening their death using a non-medical model. Thus the Caring Friends program evolved and grew.

In late 1998 the first group of Caring Friends Volunteers was trained; by 2003 there were almost 150 Caring Friends who work personally with members who have been accepted into the program. Medical records are reviewed and it is ascertained that they are capable of self-deliverance. The Volunteer is present if the member chooses to hasten her death to provide information, support, and a moral presence. It is a program of community-supported dying run through Hemlock headquarters in Denver.

Though patterned on the model started by the Rev. Mero in Seattle, Caring Friends differs from it in that it serves only Hemlock members. Volunteers will go anywhere in the country to work with a member, non-medical means are recommended since barbiturates are difficult to obtain. Another difference is that members with non-terminal but irreversible physical illnesses that have severely compromised their quality of life are eligible for the program.

Both programs—Compassion in Dying and Caring Friends—stay within the law. They do not provide the means; neither do they provide physical assistance since both these would violate the prohibition against assisted suicide. There is no charge for their services.

In France, certain groups around the country were starting to offer confidential assistance in dying (French law can be particularly punitive on occasions), while in Australia Dr. Philip Nitschke began to hold 'euthanasia clinics' around the nation to which all were invited. The Swiss have permitted assisted suicide (and not just by doctors) since 1941. In 1999, the last year an official count was taken and made public, there were a total of 1,350 suicides in Switzerland, with a mere 105 of these assisted by right-to-die groups. Ninety-nine persons threw themselves in front of railway trains that year. The government estimates that about 30,000 people attempt suicide every year, with some half of these needing extensive hospital care afterwards. Thus the amount of suicides due to mental health problems, mainly depression, very much outweighs the tiny amount of terminally ill who choose this route. The overpowering taboo on suicide in the Western world means very little is done to stem or even count the tide of self-destruction.

The Compassion In Dying idea was to begin to listen more closely to the calls for help from dying patients, or their families, and make an assessment of the sufferer's medical condition, psychological needs, pain management, and whether there was total family support. Sometimes the circumstances, such as being permanently in hospital or surrounded with a family divided on the ethics of euthanasia, meant that the request to help was declined. Alternatives such as hospice or mental health care might be advised as substitutes.

It has long been an article of faith in the progressive wings of the right-to-die movement that a person carrying out a rational suicide should not have to be alone at the time. (Of course, a few people wish to be alone.) The movement would do its utmost to provide an experienced person to sit with the patient as he or she self-delivered. Where lethal drugs were hard to come by, helium gas purchased by a member from a toy store was generally used to induce painless death within a few minutes. (This technique is explained in *Final Exit*, 3rd edition.)

It was—and is—the complete opposite of Dr. Kevorkian's tactics, which his enemies have more viciously labeled 'antics' or 'circus.' One thing Kevorkian's way did teach the movement was that even if law enforcement authorities get wind of an assisted suicide in justifiably merciful circumstances, with family assent, they may not bother to investigate. Caring Friends and Compassion keep silent about whom and where they help. Additionally, most of the pro-life groups are not vehemently against assisted suicide provided it is not made the *law* of a country with a Judeo-Christian tradition. (In 2005, Caring Friends changed its name to the more business-like 'Client Services' operating out of Compassion & Choices offices in both Denver and Portland. The grassroots of the movement became ever more baffled at the constant reshuffling.)

Guidance to Doctors

In Oregon, where physician-assisted suicide was legal from 1998 onwards, some patient services were provided by Compassion of Dying of Oregon.

(Although the way it should be carried out was minutely specified in the new law, ordinary folk and even doctors new to the procedure, often needed guidance). It is only in Oregon (Netherlands excepted) that an official count is kept of the cases and their backgrounds. But no identities can be revealed by law.

How many dying people each year are helped on their way covertly by these visiting assistants or family members? There can be no official statistics in the circumstances, of course. My estimate based on questioning and listening is that about two hundred cases happen a year in both the USA and Canada. Judging from Switzerland's experience, it is probably much higher.

Beware of whom you trust with your views on euthanasia.

For instance, a man in Northern California dying of esophageal cancer decided that he wished to hasten his end. Looking at all his options, the man enrolled in hospice, joined Hemlock's Caring Friends program, and read *Final Exit* thoroughly. He decided on the helium-bag method of self-deliverance on his own.

In the days before the week-end in which he planned his exit, he became friendly with a kind hospice nurse, and in an unguarded moment of conversation mentioned that he planned to die shortly by his own hand. Dutifully, the nurse reported his intention to her superiors at hospice headquarters. Their response was one of shock. They immediately contacted the local sheriff's department with this information.

Within minutes two deputy sheriffs turned up at the man's front door asking who had committed suicide. They were told that nho one had done so, and they left. Now alarmed at the intrusion and possible foiling of his plan, instead of waiting for the week-end, the 63-year-old man took his life immediately. He died within ten minutes, his daughter estimated. She had been present along with her mother.

A great many hospice workers are sympathetic to justified suicide and assisted suicide, and have the decency not to interfere. The working rules of many hospices say that the nurse, social worker, or volunteer, stand aside in such cases and only provide help which is not connected to the hastened death. It is not a good idea to confide any plans for a hastened death to hospice people.

It's wise also not to speak of your membership in ERGO or any other right-to-die group, or even a far-off, hazy plan for self-deliverance, to any mental health professional. They might in some cases report your thoughts to higher authority, which could order a 72-hour hospitalization in a mental ward while the case is assessed. It has happened.

Freedom of choice in how one dies should be made legal, and skilled assistance available for those who want it, though there is not—and unlikely ever to be—a consensus of public opinion on this. Like the fights state by state for Living Wills in the 1970s and 1980s, the same sort of bitter controversies are about to be repeated. It need not happen if we at least have tolerance of each other's views.

CHAPTER 11

Action for the future.

When we look at what the right-to-die movement in North America has achieved, against what it has wished to do, an honest person would agree that there is still a long, long way to go. In the 1980s and 1990s there was enormous public interest in euthanasia (see Definitions, page x) and law reforms seemed certain. But only in the American state of Oregon did a physician-assisted law slip through—and that is continually fighting not to be repealed.

Now, at the beginning of the new century, people have mostly made up their minds whether or not they support euthanasia. Prior to the 1970s, many had not even heard of the words euthanasia, assisted suicide, Living Wills, Advance Directives and so forth.

The monumental ignorance which had turned into the blazing public controversy of the previous two decades has faded.

Hail Hi-tech Medicine

Looking back, the first signs of organized activity on this issue came in the late 1930s in Britain, followed in the same decade by America, but nothing really happened until the 1970s when the public—the non-medical world—woke up with a shock to the fact that we often die differently nowadays compared to our ancestors. The medical profession could, literally, with sophisticated equipment, make a corpse seem alive with the exception of the brain. Hi-tech medicine had arrived.

This revelation—first made famous and characterized by the 'Karen Ann Quinlan pull-the-plug case in America'—brought a rush of legislation introducing the so-called "Living Wills"—better known nowadays as Advance Directives, permitting the disconnection—or declining the use of—pointless, life-support equipment.

Today Advance Directives are available, respected, pretty well everywhere in developed countries. That fight has largely been won, although the problem remains in getting people to appreciate their significance and sign them early enough before terminal ill health or a bad accident hits them.

Living Wills continually need to be improved to keep pace with medical advances and updated by the signatories, even young people. There is also a need now for a Living Will for people who may develop senile dementia or Alzheimer's Disease. Appropriate documents are now being developed in America and Europe. (ERGO has such a document.)

Where we have even further—much further—to go is related to active voluntary euthanasia and assisted suicide for the terminally ill adult, and the hopelessly ill person.

So far only the Netherlands and Belgium allow the first and second procedures, whilst Switzerland and Oregon legally permit only assisted suicide. In Switzerland it can be practiced by anyone acting altruistically, but in Oregon only by doctors. All procedures mentioned here have strong rules and guidelines built in to prevent abuse.

Elsewhere, actually helping people who desire a hastened death so as to avoid further suffering has a long fight ahead of it. There is stiff opposition. The underlying taboo in social life and the opposition of religious leaders in the rest of the Western world is holding back progress despite the knowledge that, at a minimum—judging by electoral votes and opinion polls—fifty percent of the general public wishes to see reform to give them an eventual certain death with dignity. Other opinion testings shows 70 to 80 percent support for law reform.

The main problem is: how do we convert the

converted into actual voters? The experience in America, the only place where actual citizens have on six occasions been asked to ballot on a right-to-die law, there are early indications that law reform will pass. Then, as the voters poise to place their YEA on the ballot paper, many appear to drawback. Except for the successful citizens ballots in Oregon in 1994 and 1997, the other four ballot initiatives have all failed.

Twenty-five state legislatures in America have rejected attempts introduce a 'Death With Dignity' law. The story is much the same in Australia. 'Right-to-die' isn't really on the political radar at all. In Britain, they are currently on their eighth (8th) attempt to change the law in Parliament. I wish them luck.

Why is that? Many excuses have been offered, but my conclusion is that because we are not yet carrying a majority of the medical and nursing professions in support of us, the public—understandably—panics. Who amongst us is brave enough to defy and upset our personal medical advisors?

Of course, not all doctors and nurses will ever support us. They are entitled to have religious and ethical differences. Yet only when we have a majority of them on our side—and boldly saying so publicly—can be assured that future law reform

THE GOOD EUTHANASIA GUIDE

will succeed. A good many medical professionals do support compassionate and justifiable euthanasia yet are afraid to say so openly until they see that a consensus of their colleagues agree.

What must we do to bring more of the nervous healing professions and their dithering clients around to our way of thinking?

We have to change the cultural climate in respect of individual choices in dying, and therefore we need to modify the social changes ourselves. Others in history have done it in universal suffrage, birth control, marriage and divorce laws, abortion rights, and so on. As the anthropologist Margaret Mead remarked: "Never doubt that a small group of committed citizens can change the world: indeed it's the only thing that ever has." Then what we must do to begin to bring about this sea change:

First, be right there, on the front line, at the bed-side, for dying people who seek our help. Help comes in many different ways, from straightforward advice (which is my specialty), skilled counseling, and crucial on-the-spot guidance of the rational suicide of a person who is dying, has fought all they could, and now wants a certain, quick release from this world.

The Dutch pioneered this 'at the home' approach from the 1970s onwards; also the Swiss groups have admirable set-ups. Non-doctor assisted suicide is often the appropriate action in certain cases. On the West Coast of America, Compassion in Dying of Washington State, successfully launched this type of personal compassion in the early 1900s, and Hemlock's 'Caring Friends' began similar work in 1999. It has recently been taken up by a new organization, the Final Exit Network, with a mission to guide people to their accelerated end if that is what they want. This kind of careful assistance, which comes in a multitude of ways depending on the patient's circumstances, is the most important path to build widespread voter confidence and trust. It takes time and effort but not only is it eminently worthwhile to be responding to another human's cry for help, it earns admiration from a widening circle. If there is one thing I have learned during my 25 years in this movement it is that most people want skilled help—or at least advice—right at the point when they are bringing about their final exit.

Secondly, if we are to eliminate the taboos and fears of abuse that some people have, we must make the subject of hastened death, assisted suicide, voluntary euthanasia—call it what you like—acceptable. We must get the subject better integrated into our cultures and everyday pastimes.

For too long, the Judeo-Christian religions have dominated ethical and legal thinking in the West.

The blame for making even commonsense suicide a taboo lies at the doors of the churches. That ban might have been good enough for social control in past centuries but it is not acceptable in the 21st century. Too many modern people think independently, even if believers in a deity, and wish to make their own choices.

Our goals will only be achieved when there is more written about the subject in an investigative and compassionate way. We need to work for the day when the modern news media will report 'right-to-die' matters in a straightforward way and not invent or wait for the 'scandal' and 'disgrace' incidents which they most love to report. Any movement has its low periods, its persons who are scorned.

In sum, we must introduce our subject more healthily into literature, media and the arts so that is as commonplace to read, watch, or listen to, in our lives as watching sporting events or monitoring political news.

At least we cannot blame Hollywood, the movie industry, for ignoring us. In the last few years there have been five major movies dealing with rational suicide, and all were appropriate and tasteful. (See Appendix D). The worry is, Hollywood may run out of material unless concerned new writers emerge with a passion for exploring suicide, as

Shakespeare did with Hamlet, his classic drama of psychological investigation.

Where are the Martyrs?

Thirdly, we need a few ordinary physicians in different countries to become involved in criminal proceedings: to have the courage to be the 'guinea pigs' and the *causes célèbre.* As politicians are nervous about the effect on their vote count of supporting our goals, then we should use the courts. But you cannot go to the courts without a defendant willing to take the heat and strain of a high-profile trial. Perhaps trials; certainly appeals. Such martyrs are a rarity.

We need a few doctors who will stand up and say: "My patient was suffering unbearably as he was dying. My patient was rational. I assisted a death upon request. I will fight in the courts for my duty so to help a patient." The right-to-die movement must get behind that principled physician with utmost moral and financial support.

Dr. Jack Kevorkian thought he was the man to shake the American medical profession into changing its attitude on euthanasia. But he failed, and some think he harmed the cause, while other disagree about that. His public relations problems in respect to enhancing the attitudes to euthanasia were that he was a pathologist and not a general practitioner, also more of a showman than a missionary. Some saw him as more of a 'media circus' performer than a dedicated campaigner. A loner not a team player. He thought that by himself he could alter the attitudes of the huge American medical profession. He grossly underestimated the respect doctors have for the law of the land, and how many of them are little more than body technicians and purveyors of pharmaceutical products. Without law reform accompanying it, they would not take the same chances with their lives that Kevorkian would. (He had neither wife nor children, was jobless, had no medical practice, owned no home. Nothing to lose except his liberty.)

Dr. Kevorkian's final objective was right but his tactics were wrong. But I give Kevorkian the credit for awakening millions of death-denying people to the very existence of assistance in death. The topic of one's own death is anathema to modern people, although they massively revel in the pain and death of others as entertainment on stage and screen.

Today Kevorkian languishes in an American prison, convicted on his own evidence of murder, serving ten years to life. At 76 he may never see liberty again. For all his courage and unswerving dedication he has paid dearly. His legal advisors have sought clemency or parole on health and age grounds. They were rebuffed. The predicament in thinking about Dr. Kevorkian is that, while legally he was 100 percent guilty of euthanizing Thomas Youk, who was dying—after all, he video-taped it—was it 'murder' in the usual sense of the term?

Usually we think of murder as the killing of somebody who wished to live—robbing them of life. But Mr. Youk was dying and wanted death quickly to avoid further suffering. His family agreed. Unfortunately, Anglo-American law makes no distinction on these grounds because the basis of the law is that "A person cannot ask to be killed." We must get this modified.

My plea is for the laws on homicide to be changed to allow somebody accused of a 'mercy killing' to at least be able to plead justification and necessity to the court trying him or her. By no means an automatic, knee-jerk excuse for such a drastic action but the chance to make a factual plea to judge and jury for understanding of the circumstances. Currently, no such evidence or witness in a judicial hearing in Anglo-America courts is permitted. In my view we should work for a wider interpretation of the laws on death and dying and not just 'assisted suicide'.

I also want to see more honest use of words

and phrases throughout our movement. In recent years there has been a obvious backing away from words like 'euthanasia' and 'assisted suicide' and 'mercy killing'. I am quite aware that this was done for political correctness, trying not to scare off the politicians and the voters. But it has gone too far; the public barely understands what we are now talking about.

By not calling 'a spade a spade'—as the English say—it is playing into the hands of our opponents, who increasingly are teasing us that we are more sinister than we say we are—lamb-talk in wolf's clothing. Speaking in euphemisms (softened speech to make the meaning less harsh) develops into muddled thinking and mistaken actions.

Fighting for the ultimate civil liberty, the right to choose to die when we wish and how we want, no matter what it is called, is our ultimate goal for Western society.

Late footnote: As this book went to press in 2005, it was learned that 'Caring Friends' had been re-named 'Client Services' and all but one of the four original founders let go. As a consequence, a new group emerged — the Final Exit Network.

APPENDIX A

A twentieth century chronology of voluntary euthanasia and physician-assisted suicide.

1906 First euthanasia bill drafted in Ohio. It does not succeed.

1935 World's first euthanasia society is founded in London, England.

1938 The Euthanasia Society of America is founded by the Rev. Charles Potter in New York.

1954 Joseph Fletcher publishes *Morals and Medicine,* predicting the coming controversy over the right to die.

1957 Pope Pius XII issues Catholic doctrine distinguishing ordinary from extraordinary means for sustaining life.

1958 Oxford law professor Glanville Williams publishes *The-Sanctity of Life and the Criminal Law,* proposing that voluntary euthanasia be allowed for competent, terminally ill patients.

1958 Lael Wertenbaker publishes *Death of a Man* describing how she helped her husband commit suicide. It is the first book of its genre.

1967 The first living will is written by attorney Louis Kutner and his arguments for it appear in the *Indiana Law Journal.*

1967 A right-to-die bill is introduced by Dr. Walter W. Sackett in Florida's legislature. It arouses extensive debate but is unsuccessful.

1968 Doctors at Harvard Medical School propose redefining death to include brain death as well as heart-lung death. Gradually this definition is accepted.

1969 Voluntary euthanasia bill introduced in the Idaho legislature. It fails.

1969 Elisabeth Kubler-Ross publishes *On Death and Dying,* opening discussion of the once-taboo subject of death.

1970 The Euthanasia Society (US) finishes distributing 60,000 living wills.

1973 American Hospital Association creates Patient Bill of Rights, which includes informed consent and the right to refuse treatment.

1973 Dr. Gertruida Postma, who gave her dying mother a lethal injection, receives light sentence in the Netherlands. The furore launches the euthanasia movement in that country (NVVE).

1974 The Euthanasia Society in New York renamed the Society for the Right to Die. The first hospice American hospice opens in New Haven, Conn.

1975 Deeply religious Van Dusens commit suicide. Henry P. Van Dusen, 77, and his wife, Elizabeth, 80, leaders of the Christian ecu-menical movement, choose to die rather than suffer from disabling conditions. Their note reads, "We still feel this is the best way and the right way to go."

1975 Dutch Voluntary Euthanasia Society (NVVE) launches its Members' Aid Service to give advice to the dying. Receives 25 requests for aid in the first year.

1976 The New Jersey Supreme Court allows Karen Ann Quinlan's parents to disconnect the respirator that keeps her alive, saying it is affirming the choice Karen herself would have made. *Quinlan* case becomes a legal landmark. But she lives on for another eight years.

1976 California Natural Death Act is passed. The nation's first aid in dying statute gives legal standing to living wills and protects physicians from being sued for failing to treat incurable illnesses.

1976 Ten more U.S. states pass natural death laws.

1976 First international meeting of right-to-die groups. Six are represented in Tokyo.

1978 Doris Portwood publishes landmark book *Commonsense Suicide: The Final Right*. It argues that old people in poor health might justifiably kill themselves.

1978 *Whose Life Is It Anyway?*, a play about a young artist who becomes quadriplegic, is staged in London and on Broadway, raising disturbing questions about the right to die. A film version appears in 1982. *Jean's Way* is published in

England by Derek Humphry, describing how he helped his terminally ill wife to die.

1979   Artist Jo Roman, dying of cancer, commits suicide at a much-publicized gathering of friends that is later broadcast on public television and reported by the *New York Times*.

1979   Two right-to-die organizations split. The Society for the Right to Die separates from Concern for Dying, a companion group that grew out of the Society's Euthanasia Education Council.

1980   Advice column "Dear Abby" publishes a letter from a reader agonizing over a dying loved one, generating 30,000 advance care directive requests at the Society for the Right to Die.

1980   Pope John Paul II issues *Declaration in Euthanasia* opposing mercy killing but permits the greater use of painkillers to ease pain and the right to refuse extraordinary means for sustaining life.

1980   Hemlock Society is founded in Santa Monica, California, by Derek Humphry. It advocates legal change and distributes how to die information. This launches the campaign for assisted dying in America. Hemlock's national membership will grow to 50,000 within a decade. Right to die societies also formed the same year in Germany, France and Canada.

1980   World Federation of Right to Die Societies is formed in Oxford, England. It comprises 27 groups from 18 nations.

1981   Hemlock publishes 'how-to' suicide guide, *Let Me Die Before I Wake,* the first such book on open sale.

1983   Famous author (*Darkness at Noon* etc.) Arthur Koestler, terminally ill, commits suicide a year after publishing his reasons. His wife Cynthia, not dying, chooses to commit suicide with him.

1983   Elizabeth Bouvia, a quadriplegic suffering from cerebral palsy, sues a California hospital to let her die of self-starvation while receiving comfort care. She loses, and files an appeal.

1984   Advance care directives become recognized in 22 states and the District of Columbia.

1984   The Netherlands Supreme Court approves voluntary euthanasia under certain conditions.

1985   Karen Ann Quinlan dies.

1985   Betty Rollin publishes *Last Wish,* her account of helping her mother to die after a long losing battle with breast cancer. The book becomes a best-seller.

1986   Roswell Gilbert, 76, sentenced in Florida to 25 years without parole for shooting his terminally ill wife. Granted clemency five years later.

1986 Elizabeth Bouvia is granted the right to refuse force feeding by an appeals court. But she declines to take advantage of the permission and is still alive in 2004.

1986 Americans Against Human Suffering is founded in California, launching a campaign for what will become the 1992 California Death with Dignity Act.

1987 The California State Bar Conference passes Resolution #3-4-87 to become the first public body to approve of physician aid in dying.

1988 *Journal of the American Medical Association* prints "It's Over, Debbie," an unsigned article describing a resident doctor giving a lethal injection to a woman dying of ovarian cancer. The public prosecutor makes an intense, unsuccessful effort to identify the physician in the article.

1988 Unitarian Universalist Association of Congregations passes a national resolution favoring aid in dying for the terminally ill, becoming the first religious body to affirm a right to die.

1990 Washington Initiative (119) is filed, the first state voter referendum on the issue of physician-assisted suicide.

1990 American Medical Association adopts the formal position that with informed consent, a physician can withhold or withdraw treatment from a patient who is close to death, and may also discontinue life support of a patient in a permanent coma.

1990 Dr. Jack Kevorkian assists in the death of Janet Adkins, a middle-aged woman with Alzheimer's disease. Kevorkian subsequently flouts the Michigan legislature's attempts to stop him from assisting in additional suicides.

1990 Supreme Court decides the *Cruzan* case, its first aid in dying ruling. The decision recognizes that competent adults have a constitutionally protected liberty interest that includes a right to refuse medical treatment; the court also allows a state to impose procedural safeguards to protect its interests.

1991 Hemlock of Oregon introduces the Death With Dignity Act into the Oregon legislature, but it fails to get out of committee.

1990 Congress passes the Patient Self-Determination Act, requiring hospitals that receive federal funds to tell patients that they have a right to demand or refuse treatment. It takes effect the next year.

1991 Dr. Timothy Quill writes about "Diane" in the *New England Journal of Medicine,* describing his provision of lethal drugs to a leukemia patient who chose to die at home by her own hand rather than undergo therapy that offered a 25 percent chance of survival.

1991 Nationwide Gallup poll finds that 75 percent of Americans approve of living wills.

1991 Derek Humphry publishes *Final Exit,* a 'how-to' book on self-deliverance. Within 18 months the book sells 540,000 copies and tops USA best-seller lists. It is translated into twelve other languages. Total sales exceed one million. www.FinalExit.org

1991 Choice in Dying is formed by the merger of two aid in dying organizations, Concern for Dying and Society for the Right to Die. The new organization becomes known for defending patients' rights and promoting living wills, and will grow in five years to 150,000 members.

1991 Washington State voters reject Ballot Initiative 119, which would have legalized physician-aided suicide and aid in dying. The vote is 54–46 percent.

1992 Americans for Death with Dignity, formerly Americans Against Human Suffering, places the California Death with Dignity Act on the state ballot as Proposition 161.

1992 Health care becomes a major political issue as presidential candidates debate questions of access, rising costs, and the possible need for some form of rationing.

1992 California voters defeat Proposition 161, which would have allowed physicians to hasten death by actively administering or prescribing medications for self administration by suffering, terminally ill patients. The vote is 54–46 percent.

1992 The Euthanasia Research & Guidance Organization (ERGO) is founded. Incorporated 501(c)(3) tax deductible the following year. www.FinalExit.org

1993 Advance directive laws are achieved in 48 states, with passage imminent in the remaining two.

1993 Compassion in Dying is founded in Washington state to counsel the terminally ill and provide information about how to die without suffering and "with personal assistance, if necessary, to intentionally hasten death." The group sponsors suits challenging state laws against assisted suicide.

1993 President Clinton and Hillary Rodham Clinton publicly support advance directives and sign living wills, acting after the death of Hugh Rodham, Hillary's father.

1993 Oregon Right to Die, a political action committee, is founded to write and subsequently to pass the Oregon Death with Dignity Act.

1993 European Federation of Right to Die Societies founded as a better means to tackle local problems.

1994 The Death with Dignity Education Center is founded in California as a national nonprofit organization that works to promote a comprehensive, humane, responsive system of care for terminally ill patients. Later renamed 'Death With Dignity National Center' and moves to Washington DC.

1994 More presidential living wills are revealed. After the deaths of former President

Richard Nixon and former first lady Jacqueline Kennedy Onassis, it is reported that both had signed advance directives.

1994 The California Bar approves physician-assisted suicide. With an 85 percent majority and no active opposition, the Conference of Delegates says physicians should be allowed to prescribe medication to terminally ill, competent adults for self-administration in order to hasten death.

1994 All states and the District of Columbia now recognize some type of advance directive procedure.

1994 Washington State's anti-suicide law is overturned. In *Compassion v. Washington,* a district court finds that a law outlawing assisted suicide violates the 14th Amendment. Judge Rothstein writes, "The court does not believe that a distinction can be drawn between refusing life-sustaining medical treatment and physician-assisted suicide by an uncoerced, mentally competent, terminally ill adult."

1994 In New York State, the lawsuit *Quill et. al. v. Koppell* is filed to challenge the New York law prohibiting assisted suicide. Quill loses, and files an appeal.

1994 Oregon voters approve Measure 16, a Death With Dignity Act ballot initiative that would permit terminally ill patients, under proper safeguards, to obtain a physician's prescription to end life in a humane and dignified manner. The vote is 51–49 percent.

1994 U.S. District Court Judge Hogan issues a temporary restraining order against Oregon's Measure 16, following that with an injunction barring the state from putting the law into effect.

1995 Oregon Death with Dignity Legal Defense and Education Center is founded. Its purpose is to defend Ballot Measure 16 legalizing physician-assisted suicide.

1995 Washington State's Compassion ruling is overturned by the Ninth Circuit Court of Appeals, reinstating the anti suicide law.

1995 U.S. District Judge Hogan rules that Oregon Measure 16, the Death with Dignity Act, is unconstitutional on grounds it violates the Equal Protection clause of the Constitution. His ruling is immediately appealed.

1995 Surveys find that doctors disregard most advance directives. *Journal of the American Medical Association* reports that physicians were unaware of the directives of three-quarters of all elderly patients admitted to a New York hospital; the *California Medical Review* reports that three-quarters of all advance directives were missing from Medicare records in that state.

1995 Oral arguments in the appeal of *Quill v. Vacco* contest the legality of New York's anti-suicide law before the Second Circuit Court of Appeals.

1995 Compassion case is reconsidered in Washington state by a Ninth Circuit Court of Appeals panel of eleven judges, the largest panel ever to hear a physician-assisted suicide case.

1996 The Northern Territory of Australia implements voluntary euthanasia law. Nine months later the Federal Parliament quashes it.

1996 The Ninth Circuit Court of Appeals reverses the Compassion finding in Washington state, holding that "a liberty interest exists in the choice of how and when one dies, and that the provision of the Washington statute banning assisted suicide, as applied to competent, terminally ill adults who wish to hasten their deaths by obtaining medication prescribed by their doctors, violates the Due Process Clause." The ruling affects laws of nine western states. It is stayed pending appeal.

1996 A Michigan jury acquits Dr. Kevorkian of violating a state law banning assisted suicides.

1996 The Second Circuit Court of Appeals reverses the *Quill* finding, ruling that "The New York statutes criminalizing assisted suicide violate the Equal Protection Clause because, to the extent that they prohibit a physician from prescribing medications to be self-administered by a mentally competent, terminally ill person in the final stages of his terminal illness, they are not rationally related to any legitimate state interest." The ruling affects laws in New York, Vermont and Connecticut. (On 17 April the court stays enforcement of its ruling for 30 days pending an appeal to the U.S. Supreme Court.)

1996 The U.S. Supreme Court announces that it will review both cases sponsored by Compassion in Dying, known now as *Washington v. Glucksberg* and *Quill v. Vacco.*

1997 Oral arguments set for the New York and Washington cases on physician assisted dying. The cases were heard in tandem on 8 January but not combined. A ruling is expected in June.

1997 ACLU attorney Robert Rivas files an amended complaint challenging the 128 year-old Florida law banning assisted suicide. Charles E. Hall, who has AIDS asks court permission for a doctor to assist his suicide. The court refuses.

1997 On 13 May the Oregon House of Representatives votes 32–26 to return Measure 16 to the voters in November for repeal (HB 2954). On 10 June the Senate votes 20–10 to pass HB 2954 and return Measure 16 to the voters for repeal. No such attempt to overturn the will of the voters has been tried in Oregon since 1908.

1997 On 26 June the U.S. Supreme Court reverses the decisions of the Ninth and Second Circuit Court of Appeals in *Washington v. Glucksberg* and *Quill v. Vacco,* upholding as constitutional state statutes which bar assisted suicide. However, the court also validated the concept of "double effect," openly acknowledging that death hastened by increased palliative measures does not constitute prohibited conduct so long as the intent is the relief of pain and suffering. The majority opinion ended with the pronouncement that "Throughout the nation, Americans are engaged in an earnest and profound debate about the morality, legality and practicality of physician-assisted suicide. Our holding permits this debate to continue, as it should in a democratic society."

1997 Dutch Voluntary Euthanasia Society (NVVE) reports its membership now more than 90,000, of whom 900 made requests for help in dying to its Members' Aid Service.

1997 Britain's Parliament rejects by 234 votes to 89 the seventh attempt in 60 years to change the law on assisted suicide despite polls showing 82 percent of British people want reform.

1997 On 4 November the people of Oregon vote by a margin of 60–40 percent *against* Measure 51, which would have repealed the Oregon Death with Dignity Act, 1994. The law officially takes effect (ORS 127.800-897) on 27 October 1997 when court challenges disposed of.

1998 Hemlock Foundation starts its "Caring Friends" program offering personal support and information to irreversibly ill Hemlock members who are considering a hastened death within the law.

1998 Dr. Kevorkian assists the suicide of his 130th patient in eight years. His home state, Michigan, passes new law making such actions a crime.

1998 Oregon Health Services Commission decides that payment for physician-assisted suicide can come from state funds under the Oregon Health Plan so that the poor will not be discriminated against.

1998 First 15 people die by making use, in its first year, of the Oregon Death With Dignity Act, receiving physician-assisted suicide. In the first year of the law, some 50 other applicants are refused as unqualified, or die inside the waiting period.

1998 (November) Dr. Kevorkian performs voluntary euthanasia on Thomas Youk with ALS, and a video of his action is shown on CBS TV '60 Minutes'. Within two days Kevorkian is charged with murder, and using a controlled substance.

1999 Dr. Kevorkian found guilty of 2nd degree murder and unlawfully possessing and administering a controlled drug. Sentenced to 10–25 years on the murder count and 3–7 years on the drug count. Launches appeal from prison.

2000 International euthanasia conference in Boston jointly organized by the Hemlock Society and the World Federation of Right to Die Societies.

2000 Attempt by Hemlock in Maine to get electors to pass physician-assisted suicide law similar to Oregon's fails by 19,453 votes: 51.5 percent against, 48.5 for.

2001 Kevorkian's appeal decision reached after 2 years 7 months. Judges reject it. US Supreme Court declines to hear it.

2001 MS victim Diane Pretty asks UK court to allow her husband to help her commit suicide. The London High Court, the House of Lords, and the Court of Human Rights, in Strasbourg, all say no. She dies in hospice a few weeks later.

2002 Dutch law allowing voluntary euthanasia and physician-assisted suicide takes effect on 1 February. For 20 years previously it had been permitted under guidelines.

2002 Belgium passes similar law to the Dutch, allowing both voluntary euthanasia and physician-assisted suicide.

2003 US Attorney-General Ashcroft asks the 9th Circuit Court of Appeal to reverse the finding of a lower court judge that the Oregon Death With Dignity Act 1994 does not contravene federal powers. 129 dying people have used this law over the last five years to obtain legal physician-assisted suicide. The losers

of this case will almost certainly ask the US
Supreme Court to rule.

2003 Recognizing that their goal of lawful euthanasia has been achieved, the Dutch Society
for Voluntary Euthanasia (NVVE) changes
its name to "Right-To-Die-NL". It renames the
so-called 'Drion Pill' as the 'Lastwillpill'.

2003 For political correctness, Hemlock Society
scraps its 23-year-old name and christens
itself 'End-of-Life Choices' (EOLC). Discusses
merger with Compassion in Dying.

2004 The 9th Circuit Court of Appeals found in
favor of the state of Oregon in its battle with
US Attorney General John Ashcroft, ruling
that a state had the right to decide itself which
drugs could be used in medical practice.
Ashcroft had claimed in a directive that
physician-assisted suicide was not a legitimate
medical practice, but he was rebuffed.

2004 World Euthanasia Conference in Tokyo
discusses and dissects the Living Wills
(Advance Directives) around the world.

2004 Hemlock Society USA is renamed End-of-
Life Choices and within months is merged
with Compassion in Dying to become
Compassion & Choices (C&C). This causes
the Final Exit Network to be formed from
the ashes of Hemlock to develop a system
of volunteer guides across America to help
dying people who request assistance.

2004 Lesley Martin in New Zealand completes
a seven-month prison sentence for the
attempted murder by morphine overdose of
her terminally ill mother. Vows to continue
to work for lawful voluntary euthanasia.

2005 USA Supreme Court decides to take the
Attorney-General's case against the Oregon
Death With Dignity law. Bush administration wants America's only physician-assisted
suicide law struck down on the grounds that
states do not control lethal drugs.

2005 Dr. Philip Nitschke, leader of ExitInternational,
holds workshops in Australia explaining
how to make a 'peaceful pill'.

2005 (March) Terri Shiavo, aged 41, who for over
ten years was in a persistent vegetative
state, finally allowed to die by removal of
life support equipment after a huge national
controversy involving the courts, Congress
and the USA President.

2005 First hospital in Switzerland, in Lausanne,
announced it would now permit right-to-die
group EXIT to come into wards to help a terminally ill adult who wanted assisted suicide.
Other Swiss hospitals may follow suit.

2006 (Jan.6) The Suicide Materials Offences Act takes effect in Australia, making it a crime to use a 'carriage service' to discuss end-of-life issues. Thus passing information about any form of euthanasia via telephone, internet, email and fax is a felony. Books, mail and personal meetings are not affected.

2006 US Supreme Court expected to rule on the validity of the Oregon Death With Dignity Act (1994) under challenge by the federal attorney-general. Between 1998 when the law took effect, and 2004, a total of 208 Oregon citizens used it to end their lives.

2006 (Sept. 7-10) 16th biennial conference of the World Federation of Right to Die Societies, Toronto, Hosted by Canada's Dying With Dignity organization. info@dyingwithdignity.ca

APPENDIX B

Seven years of physician-assisted suicide in Oregon.

The Death With Dignity Act was passed in Oregon by voter initiative 51–49 percent in 1994. Implementation was delayed by court actions until November 1997. The same month a second voter initiative calling for its repeal was defeated 60–40 percent. Essentially, the law became operative on the first day of 1998.

The Act permits a terminal patient with an estimated less than six months to live to ask the treating physician, first orally, then in writing, for a lethal overdose with which to end his/her life. If the physician is willing, a second physician must also examine the case and sign off on the prognosis. Should clinical depression be suspected, a mental health professional must be consulted and a lethal prescription cannot be written until or unless the patient is no longer depressed. The physician also has to seek alternatives, such as better palliative care and hospice, before proceeding. Full documentation must be kept. No health professional or worker need participate if ethically opposed to the procedure.

Residency in the state of Oregon is required. This is defined as being a property owner or renter, or having an Oregon driving license, or being on the voter's rolls.

A 17-day waiting period is mandatory. Euthanasia (direct injection) is banned. All cases must be reported to the state health department, which, at the end of each year must publish the statistics but not reveal the patient's identities. Death certificates—which are public documents—can reflect the cause as the underlying illness but not suicide.

Between 1998 to 2004, 208 patients used the law for assisted suicide out of a total of 67,706 recorded deaths in Oregon during that period. Only 13 did not die at home. In 2004 there were 37 hastened deaths — a slight drop over the previous year. Doctors were present at the bedside in six of that year's cases, and 40 had been present throughout the life of the law. In other cases mostly a trained volunteer would be present, although in 22 cases the patient ended their life without any experienced person present.

The time between ingestion of the prescribed lethal dose of either pentobarbital or secobarbital and death were a median of 25 minutes, with a range of four minutes to 48 hours.

The most likely reasons for choosing assisted suicide were, in order of importance:

1. Losing autonomy;
2. Decreasing participation in activities;
3. Losing control of bodily functions;
4. Burden on family, friends and caregivers;
5. Inadequate pain management;
6. Financial implications of treatments.

The percentage of patients referred to a specialist for psychological evaluation beyond that done by a hospice team has declined over the past seven years, dropping from 31 percent in 1998 to 5 percent in 2004.

By sex, the number of patients was fairly even — 108 men to 100 women. The median age was 69. Of the total, five were Asian and none African-American.

During the seven years, 178 of the patients were enrolled in hospice at thetime of their hastened deaths.

More detailed statistics are available at:
www.ohd.hr.state.or.us/chs/pas/ar-index.cfm

APPENDIX C

Select bibliography of right-to-die books

There has been such a rash of books dealing with this subject in the past 20–30 years that it would be near impossible to list them all. Thus I have those I believe to be most significant, and separated into different categories for easier selection.

Case histories

Death of a Man, by Lael Wertenbaker
(Random House 1975)

Jean's Way, by Derek Humphry
(Horizon Press 1978, currently in paperback)

Last Wish, by Betty Rollin
(Warner 1987; currently in paperback)

A Chosen Death, by Lonny Shavelson MD
(Simon & Schuster 1995)

How To and Advisory

Final Exit: The Practicalities of Self-Deliverance and Assisted Suicide, by Derek Humphry (Hemlock 1991, currently in paperback from Delta)

Suicide and Attempted Suicide: Methods and Consequences, by Geo Stone (Carrol & Graf 1999)

Final Acts of Love: Families, Friends and Assisted Dying, by Stephen Jamison (Putnam 1996)

Angels of Death: Exploring the Euthanasia Underground, by Roger S. Magnusson (Yale 2002)

What Dying People Want: Practical Wisdom for the End of Life, by David Kuhl, MD (Public Affairs 2002)

Fixin' to Die: A Compassionate Guide to Committing Suicide or Staying Alive, by David Lester (Baywood 2003)

History

The Right To Die: Understanding Euthanasia, by Derek Humphry and Ann Wickett (Harper & Row 1986)

Death By Choice, by Daniel C Maguire (Schoken Books 1975)

Deathright: Culture, Medicine, Politics, and the Right to Die, by James M. Hoefler (Westview Press 1994)

Freedom To Die: People, Politics and the Right to Die Movement, by Derek Humphry and Mary Clement. (St.Martin's Press 1998)

A Merciful End: The Euthanasia Movement in Modern America, by Ian Dowbiggin (Oxford 2003)

Dying Right: The Death With Dignity Movement, by Daniel Hillyard and John Dombrink (Routlege 2001)

Hospice or Hemlock? Searching for Heroic Compassion, by Constance E Putnam (Praeger 2002)

History of Suicide: Voluntary Death in Western Culture,
by Georges Minois (Johns Hopkins 1999)

The Right to Die Debate: A Documentary History,
edited by Marjorie B. Zucker
(Greeenwood Press 1999)

*Merciful Release: The History of the British Euthanasia
Movement*, by N.D.A.Kemp (Manchester 2002)

Ethics

Morals and Medicine, by Joseph Fletcher
(Beacon Press 1954)

The Savage God, by A.Alvarez (Bantam Books 1976)

Rethinking Life and Death, by Peter Singer
(St. Martin's Press 1995)

The End of Life: Euthanasia and Morality,
by James Rachels (Oxford 1986)

*Matters of Life and Death: Making Moral Theory Work
in Medical Ethics and the Law*, by David Orentlicher
(Princeton 2001)

Is There a Duty to Die? by John Hartwig et al
(Routlege NY 2000)

*The Right to Die With Dignity: An Argument in Ethics,
Medicine and Law*, by Raphael Cohen-Almagor
(Rutgers 2001)

Writings on an Ethical Life, by Peter Singer (Ecco 2001)

A Time to Die: The Place for Physician Assistance,
by Charles F. McKhann, MD (Yale 1999)

Physician Assisted Suicide: Expanding the Debate,
edited by Margaret P. Battin, Rosamond Rhodes,
and Anita Silvers (Routlege 1998)

Can We Ever Kill? An Ethical Inquiry,
by Robert Crawford (Fount 1991)

Culture

Leaving You: The Cultural Meaning of Suicide,
by Lisa Lieberman (Ivan R.Dee 2004)

Last Rights: The Struggle Over the Right To Die,
by Sue Woodman (Perseus 2001)

In the Arms of Others: A Cultural History of the Right-to-Die Movement in America, by Peter G. Filene
(Ivan R.Dee 1998)

Life's Dominion: An Argument About Abortion, Euthanasia, and Individual Freedom,
by Ronald Dworkin (Knopf 1993)

The Enigma of Suicide, by George Howe Colt
(Summit 1991)

Law

Lethal Judgments: Assisted Suicide and American Law,
by Michael Urofsky (UP Kansas, 2000)

Euthanasia, Clinical Practice and the Law, edited by
Luke Gormally (Linacre Centre, 1994)

Elder Suicide

Commonsense Suicide: The Final Right,
by Doris Portwood (Dodd Mead 1978)

Suicide in the Elderly, by Nancy J Osgood
(Aspen 1985)

Suicide and the Older Adult, edited by Antoon
A.Leenaars et al (Guilford 1992)

Suicide in Later Life, by Nancy J Osgood
(Lexington 1992)

Religion

Euthanasia and Religion, by Gerald A Larue,
(Hemlock Society 1985)

*A Noble Death: Suicide & Martyrdom Among
Christians and Jews in Antiquity,* by Arthur J. Droge
and James D. Tabor (HarperSanFrancisco 1992)

What Does the Bible Say About Suicide?
by James T. Clemons (Fortress 1990)

Playing God: 50 Religions' Views on Your Right to Die,
by Gerald A Larue (Moyer Bell 1996)

Drama

Whose Life Is It Anyway? by Brian Clark (Avon 1980)

Is This The Day? by Vilma Hollingberry
(Hemlock Society 1990)

Fiction

Moral Hazard, by Kate Jennings (Fourth Estate 2002)

Lethal Dose, by Stephen Snodgrass (ICAM 1996)

Critical Care, by Richard Dooling (Morrow 1992)

The Woman Said Yes, by Jessamyn West
(Harcourt Brace Jovanovitch 1976)

In the Night Season, by Christian Barnard
(Prentice Hall 1978)

One True Thing, by Anna Quindlen
(Random House 1994)

A Stone Boat, by Andrew Solomon
(Faber and Faber 1994)

Amsterdam, by Ian McEwan (Vintage 1999)

Stone Water, by Barbara Snow Gilbert (Dell 1996)

Mercy, by Jodi Picoult (Pocket Books 1996)

Burials and Ceremonies

Dealing Creatively With Death: A manual of death education and simple burial, by Ernest Morgan
(Barclay House, many editions)

APPENDIX D

Films dealing with dying and euthanasia

* *Based On A True Story*

Dark Victory (1939)—Bette Davis, Geraldine Fitzgerald, George Brent, Humphrey Bogart, Ronald Reagan (dir. Edmund Goulding)
Socialite who is dying gets help from a doctor. Remade for TV as *Stolen Hours* (1976).

On Borrowed Time (1939)—Lionel Barrymore, Cedric Hardwicke, Beulah Bondi (dir. Harold S. Bucque)
Comedy about an old man who isn't ready to die.

Pride of the Yankees (1942)—Gary Cooper, Teresa Wright, Babe Ruth. (dir. Sam Wood)
Classic account of life and dying of baseball star Lou Gehrig with ALS.

An Act of Murder (1948)—Frederic March, Florence Eldridge (dir. Michael Gordon)
Judge who kills terminally ill wife faces trial in his court.

The Eddy Duchin Story (1956)—Tyrone Power, Kim Novak, Victoria Shaw, James Whitmore, Rex Thompson (dir. George Sidney)
Society piano player is dying of leukemia.

On the Beach (1959)—Gregory Peck, Ava Gardner, Fred Astaire, Anthony Perkins (dir. Stanley Kramer)
Australians await death from nuclear fallout.

The Bramble Bush (1960)—Richard Burton, Barbara Rush (dir. Daniel Petrie)
Doctor in love with dying friend's wife.

Love Story (1970)—Ali MacGraw, Ryan O'Neal (dir. Arthur Hiller)
Boy falls in love with girl: girl dies.

Brian's Song (1971)—James Caan, Billy Dee Williams (dir. Buzz Kulik)
Story of Brian Piccolo, Chicago Bears footballer dying of cancer.

Harold and Maude (1971)—Ruth Gordon, Bud Cort, Vivian Pickles, Ellen Geer (dir. Hal Ashby)
The cult black comedy of a 20-year-old man obsessed with death, and his relationship with 79-year-old woman.

Soylent Green (1973)—Charlton Heston, Joseph Cotton, Edward G. Robinson, Leigh Taylor-Young, Chuck Connors (dir. Richard Fleischer)
Central theme is the "Greenhouse effect", but it contains the classic scene of Robinson's idyllic euthanasia.

Sunshine (1973)—Brenda Vaccaro, Christina Raines, Cliff DeYoung (dir. Joseph Sargent)
Couple and their doctor debate the way the wife is dying.

Murder or Mercy? (1974)—Melvin Douglas, Mildred Dunnock (dir. Harrey Hart)
Court room drama of mercy-killing.

*Babe (1975)—Susan Clark, Alex Karras (dir. Buzz Kulik)
Story of athlete Babe Didrikson Zaharias's life and dying.

*Death Be Not Proud (1975)—John Savage, Patricia Neal, Claude Akins, Mark Hamill (dir. James Goldstone)
From John Gunther's book about the dying of his 17 year old son from a brain tumor.

The Gathering (1977)—Edward Asner, Maureen Stapleton, Lawrence Pressman (dir. Randal Kleiser)
Father assembles dysfunctional family for last Christmas gathering before he dies.

*A Love Affair: The Eleanor and Lou Gehrig Story (1977)—Edward Herrmann, Blythe Danner (dir. Fielder Cook)
Story of the baseball star who gave his name to the disease ALS.

First You Cry (1978)—Mary Tyler Moore,
Anthony Perkins, Florence Eldridge, Jennifer
Warren (dir. George Schaefer)
Betty Rollin's fight with breast cancer.

Little Mo (1978)—Glynnis O'Connor, Michael
Learned, Anne Baxter (dir. Daniel Haller)
Story of tennis star Maureen Connelly's early
death.

The End (1978)—Stars Burt Reynolds as a man
who discovers that he has an incurable disease
and decides to take his own life. The bulk of this
darkly comedic film concerns his attempts to find
a painless and foolproof way to kill himself aided
by a mental patient played by Dom DeLuise.

Promises in the Dark (1979)—Kathleen Beller,
Marsha Mason, Ned Beatty (dir. Jerome Hellman)
Young girl with cancer has compassionate doctor.

Act of Love (1980)—Ron Howard, Robert Foxworth
(dir. Jud Taylor)
Man shoots crippled brother and is acquitted at trial.

The Shadow Box (1980)—Joanne Woodward,
Christopher Plummer, James Broderick,
Ben Masters, Melinda Dillon (dir. Paul Newman)
Three terminally ill patients spend a day in
discussion at a rustic retreat.

A Matter of Life and Death (1981)—Linda Lavin, Tyne Daly, Salome Jens, Gail Strickland
(dir. Russ Mayberry)
Story of Joy Ufema, crusading nurse who modernised ways of treating the terminally ill.

On Golden Pond (1981)—Henry Fonda, Katharine Hepburn, Jane Fonda, Doug McKeon
(dir. Mark Rydell)
The psychological problems of terminal old age. Henry Fonda and Hepurn won Oscars for their performances.

Whose Life Is It Anyway? (1981)—Richard Dreyfuss, John Cassavetes, Christine Lahti, Bob Balaban, Kenneth McMillan, Kaki Hunter (dir. John Badham)
Significant story of seriously injured artist fighting for disconnection from life-support equipment.

Six Weeks (1982)—Dudley Moore, Mary Tyler Moore, Katharine Healy (dir. Tony Bill)
Tearjerker about the dying of a six-year-old girl.

Right of Way (1983)—Bette Davis, James Stewart (dir. George Schaefer)
Elderly couple choose death by car exhaust.

An Early Frost (1985)—Gena Rowlands, Ben Gazzara, Aidan Quinn (dir. John Erman)
Emmy-award winning script about son who tells his parents that he is gay—and dying of AIDS.

Do You Remember Love (1985)—Joanne Woodward, Richard Kiley, Geraldine Fitzgerald
(dir. Jeff Bleckner)
Much-praised story of college professor with Alzheimer's Disease.

The Ultimate Solution of Grace Quigley (1985)—Katharine Hepburn, Nick Nolte
(dir. Anthony Harvey)
Black comedy of New York seniors employing a mafia hit man to kill them quickly.

When The Time Comes (1987)—ABC TV. Brad Davis, Bonnie Redelin (prod. Sherry Lansing)
Fictional but well-portrayed assisted suicide of dying woman.

Murder or Mercy? (1987)—NBC TV. Robert Young. Story of Roswell Gilbert's mercy-killing of his wife who had Alzheimers.

The Right To Die (1987)—NBC TV. Racquel Welch. Woman with ALS wants disconnection from life support.

Longtime Companion (1990)—PBS American Playhouse. Campbell Scott. Bruce Davison, Patrick Cassidy (dir. Norman René)
Moving and witty script by playwright Craig Lucas depicting the growth of AIDS among gay men in New York. Davison nominated for Oscar for Best Supporting Actor.

A Woman's Tale (1991)—Sheila Florance
(dir. Paul Cox)
Australian drama about 78-year-old woman
afflicted with cancer who is determined to have "a
good death." (Florance died from her cancer two
days after winning Australian Academy Award.

Dying Young (1991)—Julia Roberts, Campbell Scott
(dir. Joel Schumacher).
A 28-year-old man dying of leukemia hires young
woman who undertakes to teach him "the meaning
of life" before he dies.

Last Wish (1992)—ABC TV. Maureen Stapleton,
Patti Duke.
Betty Rollin's story of assisting her mother's suicide.

The Switch—Gary Cole as Larry McAfee, a man
paralyzed and dependant on a ventilator. Angry
and frustrated with a system that drained him of
his insurance money and leaves him in one nursing
home after another, he sues for the right to have a
switch installed on his ventilator that will allow
him to turn the machine off. He wins that "right".
This is an unusually complex (for TV) portrayal of
the issues of disability and "quality of life".

My Life (1993)—Michael Keaton, Nicole Kidman.
(dir.Bruce Joel Rubin)
Dying man videotapes his last days.

New Age (1994)—Judy Davis, Peter Weller. Complex story of self-deliverance and assisted suicide between two thirty-something "yuppies". Terminal illness is not the cause but rather their exhaustion of life's illusions.

The Last Supper (1994)—Chris (Ken McDougall) is a dancer dying of AIDS. He has chosen euthanasia to end his suffering. With the assistance of his lover Val (Jack Nicholson) and his doctor (Daniel MacIvor), he surrounds himself in his last hours with everything that made his life special and creates his ultimate work of art by choreographing his own death.

The English Patient (1996)—This Oscar Best Picture film directed by Anthony Mingella is a magnificent movie of love and war, starring Ralph Fiennes, Kristin Scott Thomas.

Particularly interesting to supporters of choice in dying is that, when close to the end of the story, the nurse quietly administers euthanasia to this dying patient at his request.

It's My Party (1996)—Directed and written by Randal Kleiser. Eric Roberts (Julia's brother) plays a man who is dying of AIDS and calls all his friends to have a party on his last night alive. Fine drama and dialogue—and it refers in passing to the book 'Final Exit'—but no one should expect to die so long after taking an overdose of drugs.

Igby Goes Down (2002)—Stars Kieran Culkin and Claire Danes, directed by Burr Steers. The main story is about a brilliant teenager who rebels and flunks out of everything. The opening and closing are remarkable scenes of two brothers helping their terminally ill mother (Susan Sarandon) to die with the aid of drugs and a plastic bag. Probably a first for showing this action in Hollywood. Rated R. 97 minutes.

The Hours (2002)—Directed by Stephen Daldry, screenplay by David Hare from the novel by Michael Cunningham. This excellent film has, as its undercurrent, the reasons for a suicide, an attempted suicide, and a rational suicide. It's the story of three women who are profoundly affected by Virginia Wolf's novel, 'Mrs.Dalloway'. Nicole Kidman won an Oscar for her portrayal of Virginia Wolf who drowns herself to escape advancing madness. Julianne Moore is the city housewife, bored and confused, who nearly commits suicide. Ed Harris plays the over-the-hill New York poet with advanced AIDS who can no longer bear to live and allows himself to fall to his death out of a window. It helps to have read the Pulitzer Prize novel first.

The Event (2003)—Directed by Thom Fitzgerald.
An intense relationship drama that takes the form
of a mystery, The Event centers around a series of
unexplained deaths that occur among the gay community in New York's fashionable Chelsea district.
Nick, a district attorney investigating the most
recent case, a suspicious, apparent assisted suicide,
and her interviews with friends and family of the
deceased trigger extensive and intricately interwo-
ven flashbacks that reveal surprising facts about
the man's life and death.

Talk to Her (2002)
Starring: Javier Camara, Rosario Flores
(dir. Pedro Almodovar)
Synopsis: Emotionally charged drama about the
intense friendship between a writer and a male
nurse who are both caring for coma-stricken
women. (Sony Pictures Classics)
Runtime: 116 minutes
Language: Spanish, with subtitles.

The Barbarian Invasions (2004)
Drama and Comedy
1 hr. 52 min.
A revisiting, some 15 years later, of the principal
characters of Denys Arcand's 1986 comedy drama
film, "The Decline of the American Empire."

Rémy, now divorced and in his early fifties, is
hospitalized. His ex-wife, Louise, asks their son

Sébastien to come home from London where he now lives. Sébastien hesitates; he and his father haven't had much to say to one another for years now. He relents, however, and flies to Montreal to help his mother and support his father. As soon as he arrives, Sébastien moves heaven and earth, brings his contacts into play and disrupts the system in every way possible to ease the ordeal that awaits Rémy. 2004 Oscar for best foreign film. Language: French with sub-titles.

"The Barbarian Invasions is a film that effortlessly makes you laugh with delight, cringe with pain and weep for life's inevitable end."
—*Chicago Tribune.*

The Sea Inside (2004)
The film focuses on the death of Ramon Sampedro, a sailor who became a quadriplegic after injuries caused in a diving accident when he was 25. After 29 years, he asked for assisted suicide and when refused, he wrote a book about his suffering, appealed to the Spanish Parliament, took out a court case, all of which failed. "I'm just a head stuck to a body," he stated. Eventually a group of euthanasia sympathizers successfully helped him with his suicide. In Spanish, with the title *Mar Adentro* and directed by Alejandro Amenabar, *The Sea Inside* won a special jury award at the Venice Film Festival, while the actor playing the lead role, Javier Bardem, won the best actor award. Opened in America in early 2005.

Million Dollar Baby (2004)

Directed by Clint Eastwood, who also acts. Highly acclaimed by the critics, who nevertheless ignore the 'message' aspect. Despite its inappropriate title and boxing ring background, the underlying theme of this film is assisted suicide and the soul-searching which precedes it. Fine acting all round.

APPENDIX E

Frequently asked questions— and the answers

Can I ask my physician for legal voluntary euthanasia (death by injection)?
No. It is against the law everywhere except the Netherlands and Belgium. And in these two nations there are strict guidelines.

Can I ask my physician for legal assisted suicide (prescribed lethal dose)?
Only in Oregon, the Netherlands, Belgium and Switzerland. All have limitation rules and guidelines.

How ill do I have to be?
The usual criteria is that a person must be terminally ill, likely to die within six months, and competent.

What if I have a protracted degenerative disease, like ALS, MS or Alzheimer's?
Doctors usually look at these case by case. The first two conditions, if advanced, are likely to get help; not so likely with Alzheimer's because the person is not in physical pain and most likely is mentally incompetent.

What is competency?
That both you and your doctor understand each other fully. An incompetent patient could not comprehend medical details.

Can I travel to any of the four places named above to get a justifiable hastened death?
Only to Switzerland. The other three have residency limitations.

Whom do I contact in Switzerland to find out if they will help?
An organization named DIGNITAS. But first write to them, at the mailing address in the list at the front of this book, outlining your needs; they have criteria.

What is self-deliverance?
Planning and carrying out one's own dying for a good personal reason. The term is a euphemism for rational suicide. 'Final Exit' is essential reading for the pitfalls and benefits of this drastic action.

Who will help me self-deliver?
Preferably your spouse or partner. Extremely rarely, your doctor. Sometimes a loyal and discreet friend.

Is suicide a crime, as some claim?
Not anymore. It never was in America but in Europe prior to the 20th century it was a crime, punishable by stripping the dead person's family of everything they owned.

Is it a crime for someone to be present or to help at a suicide?

It is not a crime to be present at a suicide. But actually helping—if the police hear about it—may be the crime of assisted suicide. It is rarely prosecuted if the circumstances are compassionate, altruistic, and there is no publicity.

Is there a group that will assist mentally ill people to die?

DIGNITAS in Switzerland will sometimes help such a case if it is long lasting, severe, and untreatable. It happens very rarely in the Netherlands. Extremely taboo subject in North America.

When was the Hemlock Society started and by whom?

In 1980 by this author, who was executive director for its first twelve years.

What happened to the Hemlock Society?

It changed its name in 2003 to End-of-Life Choices because its main mission now is law reform via politics. In 2004 it merged with Compassion in Dying to become 'Compassion and Choices.'

What is the Final Exit Network?

The Network, commenced in 2004, is building a network of 'guides' across America to come promptly to the assistance of the dying and hopelessly ill who request their support. 1-800-524-3948.

Should I sign a Living Will?
Yes, the one for your particular state or nation.
USA Advance Directives (as they are known) can
be obtained from Last Acts Partnership (see list at
front). Advance Directives indicate whether or not
you wish to be put on, or remain, with artificial life
support systems if your condition is hopeless. Give
copies to your doctor, lawyer and adult offspring.

Will my Advance Directive by obeyed by doctors?
While not legally enforceable, such documents
are a significant indication to doctors of your end-
of-life wishes. Give it to your own doctor well in
advance and ask him or her directly if it will be
taken into account. Any hesitation, change doctors.

**If I deliberately bring my life to an end because of
unbearable suffering, will my God condemn me?**
If you are an evangelical Christian, then hastened
death is a sin and therefore not an option. On the
other hand, if you feel your God is one of love,
charity, and tolerance, then He would understand
your reasons. It all depends on one's individual
faith—or lack of it—plus personal ethics.

APPENDIX F

Medical doctors accused of euthanasia in the U.S.A.

Eleven doctors were charged in the 20th century with euthanasia or assisted suicide of patients. However, none has gone to prison except Dr. Jack Kevorkian.

1935 A general practitioner in Montevista, Colorado, Harold Blazer, was accused of the murder of his 30-year-old daughter, Hazel, a victim of cerebral spinal meningitis. Evidence was given that she had the mind of a baby and her limbs were the size of a 5-year-old. Dr. Blazer, together with his wife and another daughter, had taken care of Hazel for 30 years. One day he placed a handkerchief soaked in chloroform over her face and kept it in place until she died. At the trial, the doctor was acquitted.

1950 New Hampshire doctor Herman S. Sanders was charged with first degree murder of a terminally ill patient, Abbie Borroto. At the request of Borroto's husband, Sanders injected Borroto with 44 cc's of air and she died within ten minutes. When he logged the fatal injection into the hospital record, Sanders was reported to the authorities. At the close of a three-week trial, the jury deliberated for 70 minutes before returning a verdict of not guilty.

1972 Long Island doctor Vincent Montemarano, chief surgical resident at the Nassau County Medical Center, was indicted on a charge of wilful murder in the death of 59-year-old Eugene Bauer. Bauer, suffering from cancer of the throat, had been given two days to live. Bauer died within five minutes of Montemarano's injection of potassium chloride. The defense argued that the state did not prove Bauer was alive prior to the injection. The jury deliberated for 55 minutes before returning a verdict of innocent.

1981 California doctors Robert Nedjl and Neil Barber were charged with murder for discontinuing mechanical ventilation and intravenous fluids to Clarence Herbert, aged 55. The patient had a heart attack after surgery to correct an intestinal obstruction and was declared hopeless. Following the wishes of Herbert's wife and eight children, he was taken off life-support systems but continued to breathe. Five days later the intravenous fluid was discontinued. Herbert died six days later. In October, 1983, a court of appeals dismissed the charges.

1985 Dr. John Kraai, an old-time physician from a small town in New York state, was charged with second degree murder in the death of his patient and friend, Frederick Wagner,

81. Wagner had suffered from Alzheimer's disease for five years and also had gangrene of the foot. On the morning of Wagner's death, Kraai injected three large doses of insulin into Wagner's chest. As Wagner's condition worsened, a nurse called the State Department of Patient Abuse. Kraai was charged with murder. Three weeks after his arrest, Kraai killed himself with a lethal injection.

1986 New Jersey doctor Joseph Hassman was charged with murder in connection with the death of his mother-in-law, Esther Davis, aged 80, who suffered from Alzheimer's disease. At the family's request, Hassman injected Davis with a lethal dose of Demerol. During his trial, Hassman broke down several times in court. He was found guilty and sentenced to two years probation, fined $10,000, and ordered to perform 400 hours of community service.

1987 Fort Myers doctors Peter Rosier was acquitted of first degree murder in the death of his wife, Patricia. Pat had tried already to end her life with a dose of Seconal, but when the powerful barbiturate did not take hold, Rosier began injecting her with morphine. The morphine was not lethal. Rosier did not then know it, but Pat's stepfather (who had been given immunity by the police) admitted to smothering her.

1989 Dr. Troy Caraccio, 33, of Troy, Michigan, was charged in Detroit with the murder of a 74-year-old woman hospital patient who was terminally ill and comatose. Dr. Caraccio gave the patient a lethal injection of potassium chloride in the presence of other medical staff. In court, the doctor said he did it to terminate her pain and suffering. Evidence was given that he was overworked and stressed by the recent lengthy and painful death of his father. Accepting Dr. Caraccio's guilty plea, the judge imposed five years probation with community service.

1990 Dr. Richard Schaeffer, 69, was arrested under suspicion of having caused the death by injection at the home of a patient, Melvin Seifert, 75, of Redondo Beach, California, who was suffering from the effects of a stroke and other ailments. The dead man's wife, Mary, 75, was also arrested. Both were released pending further investigation, and a year later it was announced that there would be no charges.

1990 Dr. Jack Kevorkian was charged in December with the first-degree murder of Hemlock Society member Janet Adkins who died on June 4. Suffering from Alzheimer's disease, Mrs. Adkins flew from her home in Portland, Oregon, to Michigan, where Dr. Kevorkian connected her to his so-called "suicide machine. " She chose the time to press a button which resulted in lethal drugs entering her body. Ten days after being charged, a court dismissed the murder charge.

1992 Dr. Kevorkian was charged with two counts of murder and delivery of a controlled substance for the October 23, 1991, deaths of Marjorie Wantz, 58, and Sherry Miller, 43. Both women were chronically ill

Miller with Multiple Sclerosis and Wantz had chronic pelvic pain. Sherry Miller used the 'suicide machine' to commit suicide, while Marjorie Wantz inhaled carbon monoxide through a mask. The judge in the case dismissed the murder charges when the prosecution was unable to prove that Kevorkian tripped the devices that killed the women.

1999 Switching from his usual technique of assisted suicide via his machine, Dr. Kevorkian performed active voluntary euthanasia on Thomas Youk, who was in the advanced stages of MS. With the agreement of Youk and his family,

Kevorkian injected lethal substances into the wrist and Youk died quickly and peacefully. When the authorities made no move to prosecute him, Kevorkian arranged a broadcast of his actions on the television program "60 Minutes" and on air challenged the authorities to prosecute him. So they obliged and charged him with murder and with illegally using drugs covered by the Controlled Substances Act. The video of the incident was shown in court and the jury, told by the judge that as the law stands today, euthanasia is murder, you cannot ask to be killed, he was found guilty of second-degree murder. The sentence was 10-25 years imprisonment and all appeals were turned down.

APPENDIX G

ERGO's Credo

ERGO is a nonprofit, educational organization founded in 1993 to carry out research into the best and legal ways of self-deliverance (suicide) and assisted suicide, and wherever possible, publish these findings for its members and supporters.

We hold that choosing to end one's life is a matter of personal responsibility; the reasons for so doing are in the very nature of humankind highly intimate and extremely complex. Therefore ERGO withholds judgments on people while at the same time asking that they not end their lives precipitately, thoughtlessly, and without consideration for others. Terminal and hopeless illnesses are the most justifiable reasons for a hastened death.

To this end, ERGO freely publishes throughout the English-speaking world a 'how-to' book called 'Final Exit: The Practicalities of Self-Deliverance and Assisted Suicide for the Dying.' In case some might think that this is a dark, underworld, cult book, we point out that the world's largest publisher, Random House, has handled all three editions in the past 12 years.

Well over a million copies have been sold in English and ten other languages. Thousands have used it to bring their painful lives to a peaceful end, and to thousands more it has been a comfort to know they have an escape route if they needed it.

We wish to see modifications to the laws forbidding assistance in suicide to allow it be done for compassionate and altruistic reasons (suicide itself is no longer a crime). Additionally, we seek that homicide laws get an extra provision so that the accused person can at least plead justification and ask for mercy, something not at present permitted.

ERGO also has been the main backer of a small, unofficial group of concerned international health professionals and lay experts called New Technology in Self-Deliverance (NuTech) which seeks to find fresh ways by which adults may end their lives swiftly, painlessly and legally without a physician's help. Their main achievement so far has been a technique to use inert gases, while the ultimate goal is to find the so-called 'Peaceful Pill.'

Euthanasia Research and Guidance Organization (ERGO)
24829 Norris Lane
Junction City, Oregon 97448, USA
ergo@efn.org
Phone and Fax : +541-998-1873
Web site: www.FinalExit.org

ERGO Bookstore
www.finalexit.org/ergo-store

Organizations purchasing 10 or more copies of books in bulk from ERGO receive a 40 percent discount.

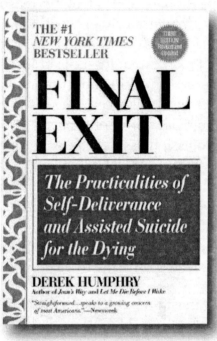

ISBN 0385 336 535

The third edition of *"Final Exit"* (in English) can be ordered at any good bookstore in the world.
(Delta Trade Paperback) *www.FinalExit.org*

From Norris Lane Press

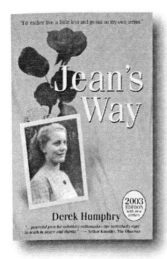

"I'd rather live a little less and go out on my own terms."

Jean's Way

Derek Humphry

2003 EDITION with new preface

"...powerful plea for voluntary euthanasia—the individual's right to death in peace and dignity." — Arthur Koestler, The Observer

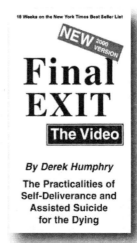

NEW 2000 VERSION

Final EXIT

The Video

By Derek Humphry

The Practicalities of Self-Deliverance and Assisted Suicide for the Dying

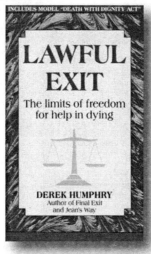

INCLUDES MODEL "DEATH WITH DIGNITY ACT"

LAWFUL EXIT

The limits of freedom for help in dying

DEREK HUMPHRY
Author of Final Exit and Jean's Way

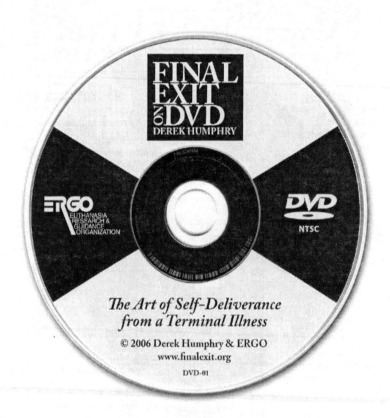

FINAL
EXIT
ON DVD
DEREK HUMPHRY

ERGO
EUTHANASIA
RESEARCH &
GUIDANCE
ORGANIZATION

DVD
NTSC

The Art of Self-Deliverance
from a Terminal Illness

© 2006 Derek Humphry & ERGO
www.finalexit.org

DVD-01

US$20